TAKE LOVE TWICE DAILY

Essays, Tales, Love Poems

Shahar Madjar, MD

Take Love Twice Daily
Essays, Tales, Love Poems
Shahar Madjar, MD

All rights reserved. No part of this publication may be reproduced, stored in a retrieval system or transmitted in any form or by any means, electronic, mechanical, photocopying, recording or otherwise without the prior permission of the publisher or in accordance with the provisions of the Copyright, Designs and Patents Act 1988 or under the terms of any license permitting limited copying issued by the Copyright Licensing Agency.

Published by: Shahar Madjar, MD

Edited by: Dr. Shai Madjar, Florence Adar, Sharon Madjar

Text and cover design by: Guy Madjar

Illustrations by: Daniel Madjar

Copyright © 2020 by Shahar Madjar, MD

A CIP record for this book is available from the Library of Congress Cataloging-in-Publication Data

ISBN-13: 978-1-7328828-1-2

Contact us at: smadjar@yahoo.com

CONTENTS

CONVERSATIONS

Ice 7

The Bet 9

The 25% Desirability Gap 19

The Art of Straightening a Banana 25

A Memorable Read 33

Love in a Rural Hospital 37

MIND AND BODY

How to Read a Poem 47

When Bud Met Mindy 49

The Princess and the Philosopher. 57

Eclipse of The Heart 61

Asleep 77

RELATIONSHIPS

Cardiology of the Bumblebee 81

Love by the Numbers 83

Folie-a-Deux 101

La Bella Luna 105

The Divorce Party 109

Collective Wisdom. 113

Please, Honey, don't treat me like a comma . 117

BIOLOGY

Take Love Twice Daily 121

The Other Girl with the Dragon Tattoo 123

Pots and Lids 131

Men are from Earth, Women are from Earth . 135

Of Mice and Men 139

Why is the Y Disappearing? 143

The Rabbit 147

Saving Romeo: Diaries of a Time Traveler . . 157

MY FUNNY BONE

Redhead 169

My Private Case of Man Flu 171

Warning Against Joy. 175

Dear Jane Loneheart, ... 179

Shall I Compare Thee to a Galaxy? 183

Newton's Apple and My Big, Red Plum 187

Acknowledgements 191

Notes on Sources 193

CONVERSATIONS

ICE

About ice
I have learned
from watching
Lake Superior.

If I drill a hole,
If I thread a line,
If I hold a hook,
Will I catch your love?

If I wear my boots,
If I hold a compass,
If I walk across,
Will I reach your heart?

If I hold my breath,
If I lean against the wind,
the snow, rain, hail,
If I wait for the spring,
for your crust to crack, for your ice to break,
Will I taste your water?

About Lake Superior
I have learned
from listening
to sheets of ice

colliding
over the face of the water
like broken glass.

THE BET

"Winter is coming," Ed told me.

"It is the middle of July and not a cloud in the sky," I reminded him.

"It is coming, nevertheless." Ed said, "This is the Upper Peninsula, and winter is always lurking behind even the brightest days."

"What difference does it make all of a sudden?" I asked.

"What good is winter if you don't have a woman to warm up against underneath a thick blanket?"

"If it's a woman you're after, Ed, shouldn't you find a woman for all seasons?" I asked.

Ed thought for a moment. "Yes, doctor, of course. An all-season woman, a year-round companion, a four-season relationship—that's what my heart desires. And it turns out, doc, that to fall in love with somebody, anybody, is a simple matter of asking the right questions."

"Questions? Right questions? Can you just tell me what is going on?" I asked.

"I read about it in the *New York Times*," Ed told me, as if sharing a secret, "a gal called Mandy Len Catron—a writer, or a reporter, I never heard of her before—she wrote an article and called it '*To Fall in Love with Anyone, Do This.*' Can you believe it, doc? It turns out that all you need is to ask the right questions, 36 of the questions, then look into the eyes of this stranger, for several minutes straight, and BOOM! Love ignites like a candle in the dark, and you fall for her, and she for you, and no more cold winters, doc."

"I doubt it. It doesn't make sense. Impossible!" I said.

"Want to bet?"

"I don't ever bet," I said.

"Why?"

"Because I hate to lose," I said.

"But you're sure that you're right, doc, right?"

"I'll make a bet with you," I told Ed, reversing my position, for I remembered the rule my father told me—that he who makes the rules, wins the game. "But only if you agree to be a subject in a love experiment."

"Now we are talking, doc. A love experiment?"

"To fall in love with anyone," I said, "that means anyone, a total stranger, a random person?"

"Exactly," Ed said.

"Here is how the experiment will go," I told Ed. "First, you will have to stumble upon a total stranger, a random person. Then ask her the 36 questions and she will ask you the 36 questions. You will then look into each other's eyes for as long as you wish. If she falls in love with you, you win the bet."

"And if not?"

"I win."

"Deal," Ed said and extended his hand, ready to shake mine.

"Just one more condition," I said. "She will have to be a complete stranger, a random person."

"And how will we guarantee she is a total stranger, a woman I found by pure chance?" Ed asked.

"Simple. We'll hang a large map of the world on a wall. We'll cover your eyes and hand you ten darts. You'll throw the darts at the map. Some darts will hit oceans and seas, but the first dart to hit a country, say Colombia, or France, would determine your destination. You'll board an airplane at an airport of your choice. There will most likely be several legs to your journey in each direction, and most likely, there would be several women that would sit next to you during these flights. Tell them about our experiment, Ed, and invite them to participate. And if you fall in love with one of them, any of them, and she loves you in return, you will win the bet."

"And who will pay for the flight?" Ed asked me.

"Whoever loses the bet," I said.

"Should I win," Ed summarized to himself, "I will have the love of my life and a free ticket to a random destination. I am so excited, doc."

"And no more lonely winters either, Ed," I said.

A map and ten darts. Ed found himself on a journey from Ironwood, Michigan to London, England. There were three flights in each direction and a total of eight women he tried to engage. And who won the bet, you wonder?

To calm my nerves, I decided to read Mandy Len Catron's article in the New York Times. I thought that To Fall in Love With Anyone, Do This is a headline that radiates authority. The story that followed was fascinating: following the suggestions of a researcher who had succeeded in making two strangers fall in love in his laboratory, Mandy applied the technique in her own life. She sat face-to-face with a man and asked him a series of questions. She reported that later, "I found myself standing on a bridge at midnight, staring into a man's eyes for exactly four minutes." Did the couple fall in love? "Well, we did," Mandy Len Catron wrote in her article.

All Ed wanted was to fall in love. And now, equipped with invaluable, scientific information he gained from Mandy Len Catron's article, he might do just that, I thought. My worries turned into despair, for I have always been a sore loser. And my heartfelt happiness for Ed's blooming mid-flight romance was mixed with bitter jealousy. But was love destined to be?

I searched for the article which inspired Mandy's "falling in love" experiment. I found it in a 1997 issue of

Personality and Social Psychology Bulletin. The principal author, Arthur Aron, was a researcher at Stony Brook University.

The study was conducted in a large psychology class. The researchers divided the students (those who were willing to participate in the study) into pairs. One group of pairs was assigned to conduct small-talk tasks. The other group of pairs was asked to carry out tasks that were expected to create self-disclosure and intimacy. The tasks, consisting of 36 questions, were to be completed in 45 minutes.

The researchers asked the small-talk group to answer questions such as: 'If you could invent a new flavor of ice cream, what would it be?' ... 'Where are you from? Name all the places you've lived.' ... and 'Describe your mother's best friend.'

The pairs in the closeness-generating group were asked to answer a more intimate set of questions: 'Take 4 minutes and tell your partner your life story in as much detail as possible.' ... 'Alternate sharing something you consider a positive characteristic of your partner. Share a total of 5 items.' ... 'Tell your partner something that you like about them already.' ... and 'Share a personal problem and ask your partner's advice on how he or she might handle it.'

How did the pairs do? Pairs in both groups—the small-talk group and the closeness group— became closer to each other; after all, they spent 45 minutes together. But the pairs assigned the closeness tasks—of self-disclosure and other intimacy-associated behavior—became significantly closer to each other (more so than the pairs in the small-talk group). It isn't just being together that made these couples closer, the researchers concluded, "the content of the tasks—whether they required self-disclosure and other intimacy-associated behaviors—made a considerable difference."

I was ready to declare defeat and admit that I had lost my bet with Ed. But when I reexamined Arthur Aron's research and read Mandy Len Catron's falling-in-love-with-anyone story again, I realized that love might be more than a random exercise in closeness, and I breathed a sigh of relief, for I could be a winner after all.

When Ed returned from London, he told me: "At the Ironwood airport, they weighed each of the passengers. The airplane was small, and the weight had to be evenly distributed so the airplane wouldn't tilt in midair. It was a single-engine Cessna with eight seats. There were only two women on the flight and no stewardess. I sat next to a Bob. I fell asleep to the hum of the propeller and woke up in Chicago.

"The Chicago flight to Paris seemed promising, from a falling-in-love perspective. The airplane was packed with people, and I sat between two women. One was a nun. She wore a stern expression and looked straight ahead into eternity. The other looked lovely, and when I started talking to her, she looked into my eyes and nodded. I told her about our bet, doc, and about the New York

Times article To Fall in Love, Do This. 'Would it be okay if I presented questions to you?' I asked her. 'We could, theoretically, fall in love. Wouldn't it be wonderful?' And she said: '*Je ne parle pas anglais.*' A bird and a fish, doc, even if they wanted to fall in love, how could they?

"The lady who sat on my right side, from Paris to London, spoke fluent English and was willing to participate in the falling-in-love project. So I asked her a question from Arthur Aron's falling-in-love experiment: 'If you could invent a new flavor of ice cream, what would it be?'

She thought for a long moment. 'Vanilla is my favorite flavor,' she said. 'It has always been my favorite and always will be.' And I immediately knew, doc, that she wasn't the one with whom I wanted to spend the rest of my life.

"In London, I did what tourists do: A walk along the Thames. A visit to Buckingham Palace. A show at the theatre. Fish and chips wrapped in an old newspaper. On my last day there, I stood on a bench in Hyde Park and argued for Brexit; then moved to the other side of the park and argued for staying in the EU. Things like that."

"What you are telling me, Ed," I said, "is that I won the bet. You didn't find love by asking a random woman a set of questions. It doesn't surprise me at all. After all, Arthur Aron—the researcher who supposedly made two strangers fall in love in his laboratory—selected students from his own psychology class, couples who shared a common background, all of the students in a prestigious university, all of them interested in psychology. These weren't random people, Ed, but people who were destined to fall in love. Even Mandy Len Catron—the woman who wrote To Fall in Love with Anyone, Do This—even she admitted that she first fell in love with a man she found suitable, and only then did she ask him Arthur Aron's questions."

"Speaking of destiny," Ed continued, totally ignoring what I had said, "I didn't fall in love—not on the flight back from London to Paris, nor on the flight from Paris to Chicago." He then stopped, as he usually does, for suspense.

"So, I win, that's my point," I said.

"But, in the Chicago airport, as I was waiting for the flight to Ironwood, I saw Susan," Ed said. "I asked her if she remembered me, and she replied that she didn't. I told her that when I fell for her, I was a junior in high school, and she was a senior. And she said she still can't remember. And I said that love has mysterious ways of uniting lonely hearts. And she asked if I was a poet. And I said that I wasn't, but I knew one. And we burst out laughing. And as we were flying back to the UP in the good old Cessna, sitting next to each other, I told her about our bet, and we asked each other the questions that Arthur Aron had composed and answered them honestly. And when we landed, we were in love, doc; we fell for each other, in midair, like love-birds.

I thought: Love is never a random exercise in closeness. In the other person, we search for the familiar, a reflection of ourselves, a projection of the ideal lover we have already formed in our mind. And yet, by asking intimate questions of each other, by responding honestly, by sharing who we are, the bridge to true love can be crossed over with greater ease.

Last week, I wrote a check to Ed. I will never bet again, not with Ed.

THE 25% DESIRABILITY GAP

1.

Six months after I had lost the bet to Ed, I met him in a cafe in downtown Marquette. Ed wore an expression of doom and gloom.

"What happened to you, Ed?" I asked. Ed wore a beret and looked like a Parisian artist on a rainy day. It was summer outside, though, and not a cloud in the sky.

"I worry too much, doc," he said, "and more than anything, it is the 25%-more-desirable theory that steals my sleep."

"How can a theory be 25% more desirable?" I asked.

"It isn't the theory that is more desirable," Ed said. "It is that scientists found that men and women pursue mates who are 25% more desirable than themselves. It was in the news, didn't you hear?"

"And how is this a problem for you, Ed?"

"I did the math, doc, and here is how it works: If Susan is 25% more desirable than I am—and she is—and if she is pursuing men who are 25% more attractive than herself, that leaves a gap of 50% between how attractive I am and the man of her dreams. It is a gap that is hard to bridge."

I told Ed: "I heard this theory before, at least a version of it. It wasn't from a scientist that I heard it, but the mother of a girl I dated. The mother wanted me to marry the daughter. There were some urgency and pressure, even desperation, in the air that hovered above the kitchen table—heavy like an ominous cloud—to marry the daughter immediately, that is. And as a measure of convincing the groom, myself, the mother said to both of us, and I remember this clearly, that for a good marriage, a man needs to be just a bit more handsome than a monkey. I suppose she thought her daughter was 25% more desirable than I was, and that this would be the key to a long, successful marriage."

"Did you guys marry, doc?"

"No," I said. "I thought she was exactly as attractive as I was, and that we were both much more desirable than the average monkey, and besides, I wanted a girl who was more attractive than me, by exactly 25%." Ed and I burst into laughter, shaking the wooden floor with our feet. I could hear the liquor bottles clinking against each other on the shelves of the cafe.

It was time for me to return home to my 25% more attractive wife, but I wanted to help Ed, so I promised I would read the article and perhaps come up with a solution that might bring calm and peace to his heart. On my way home, I walked along Third Street, then took Washington Street all the way down the hill to the lakeshore, and I continued north along the shore. The lake was calm, and the sky was bright and intense; crows seemed to be talking amongst themselves, consoling each other, about love lost. And all that time I thought about Ed and his quest for love. I thought about the men and women I know, most of whom pursue partners who resemble themselves. And I thought about those who see love as a competition in which there are winners—the popular kid in high school, the handsome celebrity, the beautiful actress—who play a part in the desires and fantasies of everyone. Doesn't that lead to the same exact result, I asked myself, where the most desirable people pair-off with one another, followed by the next most desirable, and so on, and everyone ends up with someone like themselves?

I thought: What if we could be objectively ranked according to our place in the hierarchy of desirability? I imagined Ed and Susan each opening their own letter with their desirability results. Suppose they are equal on the desirability scale, say both at the 78th percentile. And what if Susan is indeed 25% more attractive than Ed?

2.

Of all the problems facing humanity, love seems to me the most complex, and therefore I was relieved when I learned that the article Ed was talking about was written by Elizabeth E. Bruch from the Department of Sociology and the Center for the Study of Complex Systems at the University of Michigan. She and her co-author M. E. J. Newman were interested in questions like 'Is there a consensus about who is desirable?' And, 'if a hierarchy of desirability exists, would it affect who would pursue whom and whether they would end up together?'

Such information used to be nearly impossible to collect. How could researchers objectively measure one's desirability? How would they know how many suitors pursue each individual, whose love was requited, and who was left empty-handed? But now the internet, and more specifically online dating websites, are a goldmine of such information. Research on data from dating websites had already shown that people tend to pursue and compete for the most physically attractive and affluent partners, while there is a tendency to seek matching partners of similar race, ethnicity, and education.

Elizabeth Bruch analyzed data from a large-scale popular online dating website. She focused on heterosexual individuals looking for a romantic relationship in New York, Boston, Chicago, and Seattle. The researchers quantified desirability by the number of initial messages a person received. Most online love-seekers received only a handful of messages. The most popular woman, a 30-year-old New Yorker, received 1504 messages, or the equivalent of one message every 30 minutes, day and night, for an entire month. To which my initial response was: sometimes, being popular is just too much work!

The researchers measured not only the number of responders but their quality (determined by their online PageRank). They found that age, ethnicity, and education level were important desirability factors. A woman's desirability drops from the time she is 18 until she is 60.

For men, desirability peaks at 50, then declines. Asian women and white men are the most desirable. For men, more education is more desirable. For women, an undergraduate degree is more desirable, while a postgraduate degree would make a woman less desirable.

Bruch found that both men and women were sending messages to potential partners who were 25% more attractive than themselves (men were sending messages to women who were 26% more attractive than themselves. Women were sending messages to men who were 23% more attractive than themselves). The chance of getting a response was also dependent on the desirability gap. Men, for example, were more than twice as likely to receive a response from women less desirable than themselves. And, in general, the probability of receiving a response markedly dropped as the gap in desirability increased.

Ed was right again, I thought. The desirability gap is real. And people are seeking partners more attractive than themselves. What if Susan is more desirable than Ed? More so, what if she *knows* she is more desirable? Wouldn't she immediately abandon ship and seek love in more attractive waters?

As I was taking my daily walk, I thought about what I would tell Ed: "Listen, Ed," I would say, "the study was done online and you live in the real world. The study participants were seeking love among people they never met, and you met Susan in real life, on a Cessna airplane that took off from Ironwood. You fell for her, the real Susan, in high school. They are still seeking love, while Susan and you have already found love in each other's arms. Besides, to me, Ed, you are both attractive enough."

Somehow, after 5026 steps, I found myself at the Co-op on Washington Street. I sat down and drank sparkling water with an advertised, yet unnoticeable flavor of grapefruit. And suddenly, I saw Susan, standing next to me holding a cucumber, two tomatoes, and a bunch of parsley.

"Are you going to make a salad, Susan?"

"You have always been very observant," she said.

"I wanted to ask you, Susan, and I know it will sound out of the blue, if not totally awkward, but how much more attractive than Ed do you think you are?"

"I will tell you, but will you keep it a secret?" She asked.

"Of course," I said.

"I find Ed to be more attractive than me," she said, "exactly 25% more attractive." And we both laughed so hard that I was afraid she will drop the cucumber to the floor.

THE ART OF STRAIGHTENING A BANANA

"I am terrified of my barber," my friend, Dr. Daniel Doom, who is a general surgeon, told me.

"And I am afraid of death," I said laughingly.

"Seriously, Shahar, if you only knew how dangerous these people have been, believe me, you would be afraid of your barber too."

"Is this another one of your riddles, Dan?"

"A challenging puzzle this time. There are four hints to this riddle," Dan said with a teasing look of mystery in his eyes. "My fear of barbers is rooted in a 'feud that took place more than a century ago.' My fear of barbers is also related to 'a French doctor,' 'a company of barbers,' and 'the art of straightening a banana.'"

I rummaged in my mind for barber memories and for terrifying barber memories in particular. I remembered the barber in my childhood neighborhood on Mount Carmel. He was short and bald, which was funny, I had thought back then, for a barber. He was a kind, always smiling man whose razor, which he applied to the back of my neck at the conclusion of every haircut, was extremely ticklish. He wasn't at all terrifying. In Marquette, it is Kevin from Classics Barber Shop who gives me a marine-style haircut that makes me feel razor-edge cool.

His shop is a museum that treasures artifacts of nostalgic value—a price list from decades ago when a haircut was 25 cents, advertising signs for long-gone hair products, and a collection of antique scissors and razors that Kevin's father, also a barber, had used at the same shop. When I sit in Kevin's antique barber-chair, my heart fills with a bittersweet longing for a past of which I had no part. He cuts my hair with confidence, his hands moving swiftly and efficiently like those of a master-surgeon. And I don't feel terrified. Not at all.

Other barbers came to my mind: the lovely Figaro from the opera *The Barber of Seville* by Rossini; and, in sharp contrast, the completely fictional but still very convincing Sweeney Todd, whose patrons died through a unique sequence of events—they sat in his barber chair; he pulled a lever; a trapdoor opened; they fell backward, sliding into the basement of his shop; on their way down, they broke their necks; then, with a steady hand and a sadistic smile on his face, Sweeney Todd slit their throats with a sharp razor; to dispose of his customers, Sweeney Todd collaborated with Mrs. Lovett, who prepared meat-pies from their fresh flesh. Visualizing this bloody scene, I quickly concluded, 'Thank God for Kevin.'

I then directed my attention to other hints in Dan Doom's puzzle. I let my imagination fly, I let it circle around the word 'French.' I could see Paris on a cold, rainy night. I could climb the Eiffel tower. I could smell a fresh baguette and feel the crunch as I bit into its crust, or I could eat a croissant on the Avenue des Champs-Élysées. And closer to home, I could see myself at Michigan House in Calumet, Michigan, where I often dip French fries in a mountain of ketchup. I then considered the phrases 'a French doctor,' and 'the art of straightening a banana.' I asked myself, 'Why would anyone want to straighten a banana?' And BOOM, I realized that I was on to something.

'By "French,"' I thought, 'Dr. Doom must have been referring to a French doctor, François Gigot de Peyronie, who, in 1743, was the first to describe Peyronie's disease.' Peyronie's disease affects 1 in 100 men between the ages of 40 and 70 years, resulting in penile curvature, or a bent penis. It is believed that the condition is caused by an injury to the penis during intercourse. The body tries to heal the injury by forming a scar. Unfortunately, scars tend to contract, and therefore the affected area becomes shorter and narrower, resulting in a deformity, or a curve, that deviates in the direction of the injured area. Men affected by Peyronie's disease present with penile pain, penile curvature, a penile plaque (hard scar) that can be felt along the penis, and sometimes with erectile dysfunction.

In some men, the condition spontaneously improves, typically over 6-12 months. Some men would benefit from oral medications, from stretching and "modeling" of the penis, or from an injection of a substance, such as collagenase, into the penile plaque (collagenase is an enzyme that breaks down scar tissue). In many other men, the curvature may persist, creating not only emotional pain, but a functional problem as well (in the more severe cases, the curvature is so severe that it makes penetration difficult, even impossible). In these men, and only after the disease has been stable for 6-12 months, surgery may be indicated. Surgery on a curved penis, as Dr. Doom alluded, is an exercise similar to 'straightening a banana.' Looking at a banana you would notice that it has a longer side and a shorter side. Straightening it would require either shortening of the longer side or lengthening of the shorter side. And that is exactly what is done during the surgery to correct penile curvature: the shorter side of the penis is lengthened by removing the plaque and adding a larger graft (like a patch), or by shortening the longer side—by making several longitudinal incisions that are closed horizontally.

I felt some relief knowing that I had managed to solve at least a part of Dr. Doom's puzzle. On my list, I added a checkmark next to 'a French doctor' and another checkmark beside 'the art of straightening a banana.' That night I couldn't fall asleep. As I was tossing and turning in bed, I asked myself, 'What the heck did Dan Doom mean when he mentioned 'a company of barbers,' and what was the "feud" that led him to fear them so much?'

The next day, I looked at a picture of François Gigot de Peyronie. I saw a serious man sitting in his library, dressed in the best garments Paris had to offer, and wearing a long, curly white wig. His expression was that of accomplishment, fame, and power. As I kept reading about the man, the reasons for his self-indulgence became evident. Peyronie was the Chair of Anatomy and Surgery at the University of Montpellier, the commander of the medical corps in the army of Louis XIV, and the founder of the Royal Academy of Surgery. So famous was he that among his patients one could count the kings of Poland and Prussia, as well as the mistress of the Prince, the Countess Vintimille. Peyronie also earned the confidence and affection of Louis XV, the king of France, after he cured him of 'a delicate disorder' in 1738.

On a cold day in February 1745, Peyronie must have felt particularly powerful, even influential, for it was on that day that he found himself sitting next to his desk to write a letter to the Lieutenant of Police, urging him to take immediate action against the barber-surgeons of France. The barber-surgeons—the predecessors of my childhood barber on Mount Carmel and of Kevin, my barber in Marquette—had a different role in Peyronie's time. They were the medical practitioners of medieval Europe, their scope of practice reached wide and deep. They served as barbers, surgeons, and dentists. Trained as apprentices without any academic degree, these barber-surgeons not only cut hair, shaved chins, and trimmed beards; they engaged in almost any other medical intervention available at the time—leeching and bloodletting, enemas and fire cupping, neck manipulation, cleansing of the ears and scalp, draining of boils, and the extraction of teeth. That was the state of affairs that Peyronie was determined to change. He wanted barbers to be barbers and surgeons to be surgeons. He wanted to draw a clear line of demarcation between the two.

'These barber-surgeons must have been the "company of barbers" that Dan Doom, the general surgeon, was talking about,' I thought.

In his letter to the Lieutenant of Police, Peyronie, the "protector of surgery," demanded that these barber-surgeons be forced to sign an agreement to quit practicing the way they had been. His words carried weight, and soon thereafter, four of the barber-surgeons were arrested and locked up in jail. They were later enlisted in the regiments of Champagne, a military unit, and sent off to battle where they had a good chance to be shot. This, according to the Lieutenant of Police, "gave great satisfaction to La Peyronie."

"I now know why you are so terrified of barbers," I told Dan. I asked him if my solution to his riddle was correct.

"Absolutely," Dan Doom said, smiling.

"Are you seriously afraid of barbers, Dan?"

"You never know," Dan Doom said, "they may still hold a grudge."

A week ago, as I was waiting in line for my turn to have my hair cut at Classics Barber Shop, I suddenly remembered my colleague, the doctor, his riddle, and his fear of barbers. I looked at the barber pole, spinning with red and white stripes, a distant symbol of the two crafts once held by barbers—white for barbering and red for surgery—and in my mind, the feud between doctors and barbers was long over. Still, just before I sat in the antique barber chair, I checked it carefully, and, to my relief, I found no trapdoor. Kevin, my barber, was cordial as ever and showed no clear signs of animosity.

A MEMORABLE READ

Sharon falls in love with her books, but not faithfully. She commits to live-happily-ever-after with one book, but later she abandons it and dates another in secret, only to return to the arms of the first book, to find comfort and solace in its pages. She is a general, commanding an army of books that occupy our home. Some books are obedient; they are standing tall next to each other on shelves like good soldiers, but others have defected from the line of duty—they lie on top of each other at different angles, threatening to fall. At times her books are an angry crowd hungry for attention. They demonstrate on chairs and sofas and on tables and desks. Yet other books are shy, quietly waiting for their turn, hiding in the bedroom upstairs, in the kitchen cabinets, and on the countertop just around the fruit plate. Whether they are non-fiction or fiction, biographies or memoirs, suspense or murder mysteries, simple stories or convoluted plots, Sharon reads them all.

Like Sharon, I read too. But I choose my books carefully. I judge books by their cover, their weight, and the size of their fonts. I like short stories in soft covers and moderately complex essays with bright, concise ideas. To prevent confusion, I prefer tales with fewer than five characters whose names and appearances are different from each other. I prefer plots in which nobody hops on an airplane and all characters stay put. I like my readings to be completed in one sitting: articles on current and past events, art and leisure, money and business, science and medicine. When I read, I tuck a pencil, fashionably, behind my ear, and at times when I feel the urge, I draw my pencil like a sword, and I mark interesting ideas, words that I did not know, and just anything I find beautiful.

The other night, I asked Sharon: "In the end, what will happen to our memories?" She stopped reading her thick book—'War and Peace,' I believe it was—and said, "write a memoir and your memories will last forever. I may read it too if I find some time."

I thought the discussion on memories was over, but the next day Sharon urgently corresponded, via email, informing me that she had just read an article that I would find interesting. "It is about memories and their preservation," she wrote.

The study, 'Life-span cognitive activity, neuropathologic burden, and cognitive aging,' was conducted by Robert Wilson and his colleagues from Rush University Medical Center in Chicago. It was published in the journal 'Neurology.'

Participants in the study were first asked about their life-long participation in cognitively stimulating activities, such as writing letters, visiting a library, and reading books. Their cognitive function (including their memory) was then measured, yearly, using 19 different tests.

Several years later, once the study participants eventually died (of natural causes, I must clarify; the authors should be congratulated for their patience), their brains were removed, and their brain tissues preserved, sectioned (I will spare you the details), examined under the microscope, and evaluated for changes typical of dementia (amyloid burden, presence of Lewy bodies).

The results were clear: "more frequent cognitive activity across the life span has an association with slower late-life cognitive decline." In other words, the more people read, the better they remember.

I tried to remind myself that statistical associations do not necessarily mean cause-and-effect relationships. But still, in my mind, I could see the droves of avid readers discussing the findings of this research in book stores and in libraries, in book clubs and in literary forums on the internet.

As for myself, and just to be on the safe side, I immediately asked Sharon for some book recommendations— longer books with multiple characters who tirelessly wander around the world in search of meaning.

LOVE IN A RURAL HOSPITAL

I learned about love mostly from listening to the stories of others. These are tales of unrequited love—of ghost towns, elephants, and compulsory anger management classes.

Dr. Jim Darkroom, a radiologist, once told me: "In the end, I just bought a ghost town for Rachel with a small town square and a church standing tall in its center. But at the beginning, some years earlier, at an Italian restaurant, in Venice, Italy, after we shared a divine tiramisu, when I knelt in front of her and handed her an engagement ring, she laughed at me, and everyone was watching as she said no. Three years later, after her mother died, her sister moved to Columbia, and she finally finished reading *A Hundred Years of Solitude*, I thought I should ask for her hand again, but, for heaven's sake, this time I should do it right. At a Celine Dion concert in Atlanta, I jumped on the stage during the intermission, grabbed the microphone and shouted, at the top of my lungs, "Honey, I love you! Will you marry me?" There were tears in my eyes, as I raised my hand in the air, holding an even larger engagement ring. Several security men rushed toward me to get me off the stage. One cameraman was projecting my image onto the big screen. Another camera found Rachel in the crowd. On a split-screen, for everyone to see, I was on the right side of the screen, my whole body shaking with love, and on the left side of the screen, she was standing, shaking her head, her lips moving in silence: "Sorry honey, but I just can't. I am so sorry." So, last year I bought a village in the Upper Peninsula of Michigan. It was a mining town, way back when people were willing to pay gold for copper. Then the demand for copper dwindled and everyone left town. There was a deserted church in the town square, a gas station with a tilted roof and a dry pump, and three empty old homes that were threatening to tumble. Here is what I will do," Jim told me several months ago when he was still working at my hospital. "I will renovate the church, paint and all. I will invite Rachel to see the place—and trust me, it will be beautiful—and with the light pouring through the colored window glass, I will kneel in front of her and ask that she marry me and live with me at the church, at the top of the hill, just the two of us alone, together, forever."

Dr. Howard Burnett, an ear, nose, and throat doctor, once told me: "I fell for Rachel, the receptionist from the main lobby—you know her, right? I took her out one night to Bob's Family Diner and tried to figure out what it would take for us to be together, as a couple—you know, right? You know. I asked Rachel if she would come with me, to New Orleans. 'I have a conference there,' I said, 'and I could take you to a jazz club.' She listens to classical music only; violin concertos, to be exact. 'A hunting trip to Africa, perhaps?' I tried again. No! She prefers riding elephants in India where she heard elephant rides are the best. Besides, she is taking classes for nursing school, and she believes in holistic medicine—she tells me one can heal an ear infection, even throat cancer, by acupuncture, and that crystals if placed at the exact position along the spine, would heal even the deadliest of diseases. She also believes in homeopathic medicine. She says that the less medicine you use, the more powerful it is. 'To any malady,' she said to me, 'the solution is dilution.' She speaks in rhymes, did I tell you? I must have. Besides, and I am serious here, she told me she had always wanted to meet the Dalai Lama. The next day, on my way to work, I was listening to the radio. On NPR they said that the Dalai Lama wasn't well, something like pneumonia. So, I arrived in my office, took off my raincoat, put on my white coat, straightened my tie, and ran downstairs to inform Rachel that time is running out, and if she wanted to meet the Dalai Lama, she should leave work right away and hop on a flight. She saw my remarks as a personal affront. 'I don't think we should see each other anymore,' she said. The next day, on CNN, I heard that the Dalai Lama was doing much better and was no longer in critical condition. Perhaps he was cured by the power of crystals."

Here is what Dr. Goldfinger, a gynecologist, once told me about Dr. Night: "Dr. Night, the ER doctor, flies in from Ohio. He works only one week a month, but when he works, he stays at the hospital around-the-clock. His voice is always hoarse because he never sleeps. His eyes are bloodshot and weary. He has the body of a mountain climber, because, on his monthly three weeks off, he finds pleasure in climbing steep mountains. He loves athletic women, he told me, who are fun to be with and have a good sense of humor. Women love him. They find him attractive, because he is good-looking, but more so because he makes short visits and then fades away into the mountains. In short, he is emotionally unavailable. In the ER, he makes swift medical decisions that are almost always accurate. I know all that because he wakes me up often, in the middle of the night, to discuss interesting cases in gynecology. I think he is just lonely.

"The other day, Dr. Night admitted an elderly man to the Med-Surg Department on the 5th floor of the hospital. The old man had congestive heart failure and had difficulty breathing. The old man responded well to diuretics, but he still looked frail and confused. Dr. Night tried to call Dr. Day, the hospitalist in charge of the 5th floor, but there was no answer, there was never an answer, so he made an executive decision and just sent the patient up. Minutes later, the nurse, Rebecca, told Dr. Night that Dr. Day wasn't happy at all with the admission and that he, Dr. Night, should go up and straighten things up.

"The conversation on the 5th floor took place in the long corridor of the department next to the nurses' station. The doors to the patients' rooms were open, and everyone could hear everything. Several nurses stood along the corridor next to their mobile EMR stations, filling in vital signs, recording patients' levels of pain. Others, inside patients' rooms, were dispensing medications, or just talking with their patients. The nurse manager was in her room trying to find a replacement for a nurse who had called in sick. The air carried the usual blend of background voices, TVs that were turned on to different stations, and the constant beeping of monitors.

"Why the heck did you admit this patient?" Dr. Day asked.

"He is elderly, frail, barely alive, and he couldn't breath. What else could I have done?" Dr. Night said.

"He is breathing just fine," Dr. Day said.

"I gave him enough Lasix to kill a horse," Dr. Night said. "He may be breathing now, but he may stop breathing in two hours, once the effect of the diuretics wears off."

"Why didn't you at least call me before you admitted the patient?" Dr. Day asked, raising his voice.

"Because you never answer your phone," Dr. Night said.

"I always answer my phone," Dr. Day said.

"Perhaps, but not when I am calling," Dr. Night said.

"I will answer your calls as soon as you stop having sex with my girlfriend!" Dr. Day shouted.

Dr. Night did not ask who Dr. Day's girlfriend was. He didn't say that he didn't know that she was his girlfriend. He didn't say he was sorry. There was silence. The ever-present hum of the hospital had turned into dead silence. The nurses along the corridor stopped typing. Other nurses came out of patients' rooms and stood at the doors looking at the two doctors. The nurse manager raised her head and took her eyes off the computer screen, wondering if what had just happened had indeed just happened. The monitors seemed to stop beeping. At that moment, it was 5:32 in the afternoon, and at the administration office, five floors below, Mrs Miller, the Chief Nursing Officer and Mrs Johnston, the CEO, must have felt that something had gone terribly wrong. Minutes later, they were called to the 5th floor. Dr. Night had left. He was back in the Emergency Room treating a woman who had hit her head on a street sign and was profusely bleeding from her scalp. Dr. Day was sitting alone in his room, his head in his hands. The floor nurse manager told the two higher-ups what had happened. There was only one solution to a development like that, they all knew, and it wasn't to fire the doctors. After all, this was a rural hospital in the middle of nowhere, where the winds blow hard and the snow piles up to the windows of the second floor, and recruitment, especially of good doctors, is very difficult. No! The solution was simpler, and it worked well, and if it were to fail, they all knew, the doctors would just leave on their own anyway. Two weeks later, Dr. Day and Dr. Night found themselves in a crowded conference room in Las Vegas. They sat at opposite sides of the lecture room, wearing an expression of reluctance and taking notes in a class called 'Anger Management for the Practicing Doctor.'"

All of that had happened a while ago, and since then, Dr. Darkroom, Dr. Howard Burnett, Dr. Day, and Dr. Night had all left our small, rural hospital and found their calling, each in a different small, rural hospital—far enough from our hospital that I have never heard from them again.

On my short breaks between seeing patients, I often walk downstairs and buy a cup of coffee at the gift shop. Mrs Rosenberg, who volunteers there, makes the best coffee in the world. Besides, she is talkative and always pleasant.

"Tell me, Doc, did you notice that many of our good doctors have left?" Mrs Rosenberg asked me as she poured hot, foamy milk into my coffee. "As soon as we get used to a doctor, he leaves the hospital for good."

"It must be the weather," I told her, searching in my pockets for change. "Also, who wants to live in a place so remote from everywhere else?"

She laughed whole-heartedly and said, "You know, Doc, I was once a psychoanalyst. I even met Sigmund Freud once, in Vienna."

"And what have you learned, Mrs Rosenberg?" I asked.

"It isn't the weather, Doc," she said, in a quiet voice. "Dr. Darkroom had left because the woman he loved wouldn't say yes to his proposals, not even in the most romantic of churches in the most beautiful of deserted towns. Dr. Howard Burnett didn't fancy any of the other local girls, and so he couldn't find love here. And Dr. Day and Dr. Night couldn't live with the idea that if they were to be with the woman they both loved, with Rachel, they would have to share her. Anger management class couldn't heal a broken heart."

"Do you have a solution, Mrs Rosenberg?"

She handed me the coffee and said, "Love is often an unsolvable puzzle, the pieces don't always fit. And, let me tell you, Doc, the pieces don't have to fit—it's the search for love that matters; it is the quest for love that gives life meaning."

MIND AND BODY

HOW TO READ A POEM

I look at your lines.
So delightful are the contours
of your hilly curves,
the serpentine turns
your scenic routes take.

I open your stanzas.
So inviting are the spaces
in your chest of drawers,
the mysterious corners
your fresh ideas form.

I read your words.
So enticing are the sounds
of your joyous melody,
the truest songs
your fine notes compose.

Remember our trip to the Grand Canyon?
I stand at the edge of a cliff,
I whisper you as a prayer,
I shout you over the void,
waiting for the echoes to call my name.

WHEN BUD MET MINDY

Mindy and Bud were on their way to meet each other in the middle of the country. She told him that she was a psychology student in New York. He was an engineering student who lived in L.A. Bud consulted Google and made the calculation: the distance between them was 2845 miles, and the middle of the road fell along I-80 in Waco, Nebraska, population 236.

There were no restaurants in Waco, but Chez Bubba Cafe in Goehner was close by and got good reviews. Besides, it was the kind of place whose name stirs the imagination with curious questions, such as "Who is Chez Bubba?" and "How did he end up in Nebraska?"

Mindy and Bud's relationship had begun two months prior. It was a Wednesday evening, and therefore Bud was working on his upper body at the gym. He followed a strict, high-protein diet and a body building program called "muscle confusion." He worked his biceps and then his triceps, his pectoralis major and then his latissimus dorsi muscles. He did pushups and lifted weights. And when he checked his reflection in the mirror, he concluded that his muscles must have been well confused and that he wasn't in bad shape after all.

Back at home, he took a shower and did his homework, answering some questions in Mechanical Physics.

Then, he sat in front of the TV and searched the internet for "building a better body." One thing led to another, and he found himself on Reddit.com, in the philosophy section called 'Mind and Body.'

A girl, Mindy, posted a question: "I am interested in the mind-body problem. I have read about it, quite a lot honestly, but I am still confused. I wonder if there is someone out there, preferably a non-philosopher, who can solve the problem in simple terms."

Bud was intrigued. He continued to read Mindy's post: "The problem goes something like this: when I play the piano, for example, my fingers move along the keyboard. This movement takes place in the physical world. Physicists and mathematicians can measure the movements of my fingers in physical terms such as how fast my fingers move and what distance they cover. Biologists can explain how the muscle cells in my fingers contract and relax. Neurologists can measure action potentials along the nerves that innervate my fingers. Radiologists can take images of my brain and show areas that light up while I am playing the piano.

"The problem is: how does my desire to play the piano and the commands my mind gives my fingers translate into the movement my fingers make? Is my mind separate from my body, and if so, where does the connection between the mind and body take place?

"And in a similar way," Mindy continued, "when I listen to music, I hear it, I experience it, I feel it! I feel sadness when the music turns melancholic and happiness when the music is joyful. Scientists can measure the sound waves, describe the mechanical properties of the ear as an instrument of hearing, measure the impulses traveling through my inner ear and into my brain, and even indicate the areas where cells in my brain are lit-up in response to sound. But how I experience music—the joy I draw from it, the emotions it evokes in me—these exist in my private world only, in my own mind.

"And the problem is," Mindy continued, "how do sound waves in the physical world translate into my experience of music? Is my body separate from my mind, and if so, where does the connection between the body and mind take place?"

Bud thought that Mindy was cool, really cool. "I think that your mind and body are one," he wrote. "I could never understand the fascination scientists have with the brain. I say: It is a substance like all substances are, made of atoms and molecules. Computers that are made of copper, lead, gold, and plastic can already win chess championships and drive automatic cars in cities and along highways. Give me time, money, and a bunch of dedicated computer scientists, and I promise to build a computer, made of atoms and molecules, that would work exactly like your brain does: it will think, be aware of its own existence, experience joy, and feel pain. It might even fall in love with you! The mind–body problem is not a problem, it is just an illusion. And, by the way," Bud added, "do you really play the piano? I would love to listen."

Over the next several weeks, Mindy and Bud continued their conversation, first on Reddit and then via email.

"I still believe in the immaterial soul," Mindy wrote, "and in the mystery our mind is. Perhaps I could convince you if we ever met."

"Dear Mindy," Bud wrote, "why wouldn't we meet? It would be an adventure. We could drive toward each other (I made the exact calculation) and meet in the middle of the road, just next to Waco, Nebraska, at Chez Bubba Cafe.

It was a summer day and the air-conditioners at Chez Bubba Cafe could barely keep up with the heat. Bud was sitting next to the window, facing the entrance door. The cafe was empty. At noon, as scheduled, he saw Mindy through the glass, arriving in a pink Volkswagen campervan from the early sixties. He noticed that she was thin, her hair was bright red, and that her stride was so delicate that she seemed to almost float in the air.

She entered the restaurant, looked around, noticed him, and approached his table. "Bud, I assume."

"Mindy," he replied, got up, and kissed her on her cheek. They sat down across from each other. The table was narrow, their knees almost touching. They talked about their long drive and the sights that they saw along the way. He ordered a steak, medium rare, with French fries. She had the portobello mushroom wrap with shredded carrot on the side.

"I thought about what we were writing to each other, about the mind-body problem," Mindy said. "I wanted to prove to you that there is a soul, a separate entity from the material body. Here is exercise number one: describe me."

"You are tall and thin, your hair is red, and, to be honest, you are cute," he said with a smile on his face.

"So, in the world according to Bud, where all things exist merely in the physical world, rays of light are transmitted into your eyes, through the lenses, and fall on layers of cells in your retina. This would cause your optic nerve to generate minute electrical currents that would move into your brain. Your brain, which is no more than a super processor made of billions of cells, would read the signals and translate them into something like: tall, thin, red hair, gorgeous," she said, "and thank you, by the way, for the compliment. I like the way you look too."

"Exactly! And thank you," Bud said.

"Here is exercise number 2: come closer to me," she whispered and leaned forward over the table, half-way toward Bud. "I want to ask you something." Bud leaned forward, his ear was close to Mindy's lips. "How do I smell?" she asked.

Bud took a breath in and focused on Mindy's scent.

"Sweet. Better than a flower in a Georgia O'Keeffe painting," he said.

"So, molecules of scent travel through your nose, activate cells in your olfactory bulb, and the message is transmitted into your brain, which calculates the smell and searches for mental images such as that of a flower in a painting by Georgia O'Keeffe."

"Yes."

"Now give me your hands," Mindy said as she extended her arms across the table, reaching for Bud's hands, "and let's hold hands and look into each other's eyes." Bud complied, of course—what else was there to do in Nebraska? Besides, there was beauty in Mindy that he had never seen before, a power in her that excited every cell in his body. "Now, tell me what you feel, whatever comes to your mind," she said.

"Your skin is warm. I feel waves of warmth radiating from you. I see kindness in your eyes, and when you are smiling at me, right now, I feel that my cheeks are warm, and that my heart is beating faster. I feel as if thousands of magnets work their way between us. It is magic, Mindy. I want you."

Three months later, back in L.A., Bud was sitting at his desk, thinking about the events of that day at Chez Bubba. He remembered going to the back of the restaurant and paying for lunch. When he returned to the table, Mindy was gone, and her Volkswagen camper-van was also gone. In the days that followed, he tried to contact her by phone and online. She didn't respond.

On Reddit, on the "mind-body" board, Bud noticed a new post by a guy called Bill who wrote: "The strangest thing happened to me. I always believed in the body and mind being one – a super-computer, nothing more. Then, I met this girl, Mindy, online. Mindy was a student at the University of North Dakota. She believed in dualism (mind and body are separate entities). She wanted to meet me about halfway, in Nebraska (I am a student at the University of Northern Texas), to further discuss the mind-body problem.

"Long story short," Bill continued, "I met with Mindy and fell for her (others call it love. I never knew what love was before I met Mindy). I always thought that the mind is only an illusion. But let me tell you, after meeting Mindy, I realized that my mind is more than the sum of the brain's components; it is more than just atoms and molecules.

"Some believe that the mind is an illusion," Bill wrote, "but even if this were true, for those of us who experience life, who let themselves feel their emotions, the mind is an illusion so strong that even when you know it is an illusion, you cannot relate to it as a mere illusion. Your mind becomes a reality.

"I lost contact with Mindy. Did anyone have a similar experience? Who is Mindy?" Bill asked on the discussion board.

Bud knew the answer: Mindy did not live in New York, nor in North Dakota. She was a local girl from Waco,

Nebraska, and she wanted everyone to know that the mind is not a mere illusion, that souls exist, that love is real. She was about to prove it all, one man at a time.

THE PRINCESS AND THE PHILOSOPHER

How can souls move bodies?

In a seventeenth century portrait, Princess Elisabeth of Bohemia looks like a princess who knows she is a princess. She sits upright and radiates confidence, her skin pale without a blemish, her curls cascading over her shoulders. She is wearing an elegant, elaborate hat and a shiny pearl necklace. She is holding a long and heavy hunting spear, but seems to have no interest in hunting. In her wise, curious eyes there is an invitation for an intellectual duel.

In 1643, the princess invited Rene Descartes to such a duel. Descartes, a philosopher known even to non-philosophers for his most quoted philosophical argument, "I think, therefore I am," agreed to the proposal. They corresponded from 1643 to 1649. They wrote more than fifty-eight letters to each other. They also met in person. In her first letter to Descartes, after reading his meditation "Concerning the Existence of Material Things, and the Real Distinction between Mind and Body," the princess became curious, and so she began writing to Descartes, presenting a fundamental question: "Given that the soul of a human being is only a thinking substance, how can it affect the bodily spirits, in order to bring about voluntary actions?"

Descartes responded the way a true gentlemen of his time would, apologizing for his inability to express his thoughts appropriately. He admitted that when they had met, it was the Princess's dazzling combination of intelligence and beauty that distracted him and prevented him from properly explaining the bodily spirits and the voluntary actions. He wrote, "I can't hide anything from eyesight as sharp as yours! My principal aim was to show that the soul is distinct from the body." In a desperate attempt to redeem himself, he compared the effect the soul has on the body to the effect the weight of a rock has as it moves the rock toward the center of the earth. She was trying to comprehend the mind-body problem; he was stuck on gravity.

The sharp-eyed Princess immediately realized that Descartes wouldn't, or, more likely, couldn't provide a good answer to the mind-body question she presented. "This leads me to think," she wrote to him, "that the soul has properties that we don't know—which might overturn your doctrine . . . " She then did what women often do when they recognize men's shortcomings, but still want to keep the conversation going—she changed the subject.

She wrote about her annoyance and boredom running the interests of her semi-royal family (her father was a king for just a short while, then lost his kingdom to the Holy Roman Empire). Descartes wrote back reporting on his voyage to Paris, which "could not involve any misfortune when I had the good fortune of making it while being alive in your memory." They discuss moral dilemmas, vices and virtues. They correspond about magnetism and the fire at the center of the Earth. They express mutual admiration and practice false self-deprecation. She tells him about her health and maladies, and he advises that the most common cause of low-grade fever is sadness. He tries to entertain her by sending geometry riddles. She solves them with ease, half-asleep, before bedtime.

In the long correspondence between the princess and the philosopher, the question of how souls move bodies is not revisited. It is not for lack of elaborate, complex theories. In his writings, Descartes extensively described the connection between mind and body. According to Descartes, the body is nothing but a machine. Its blood and its spirits are agitated by the heat of the fire continuously burning in the heart. And the pineal gland is the place where all of our thoughts are formed and where the soul is immediately joined to the body. Descartes' ideas are so wrong, they would have never passed the scrutiny of a sharp-eyed princess.

In 1649, Descartes accepted an invitation from Queen Christina of Sweden to visit her castle and to give her lessons in philosophy. He writes to the princess that the Queen "has as much merit as she is reputed to possess, and more virtue." The Princess of Bohemia writes back that she is not at all jealous by Descartes' affection for the Queen.

It was winter in Sweden. The Queen insisted on taking her philosophy lessons early in the ice-cold mornings. The philosopher, unaccustomed to rising early, nor to the harsh winters, caught a cold and, at the age of 53, died of pneumonia. The fate of Descartes' bodily remains poetically fits his philosophical, dualistic views of the mind and body. He was buried in Stockholm, Sweden. His body was then exhumed, taken to France, buried, exhumed again, and buried again, missing a forefinger and the skull, in the Abbey of Saint Germain-des-Pres.

The National Museum of Natural History in Paris claims to hold the philosopher's skull.

ECLIPSE OF THE HEART

1.

Sometimes I wonder what it would be like to live in a different time. I have no desire to live in the trenches during a world war or to lead a revolution, nor do I want to live through famine, earthquakes, or a global flu epidemic. Instead, I want to return to those moments in which ideas that were born in creative minds finally came to fruition. Take me back to the day on which Anton Chekhov finished writing *The Lady with the Dog in her Lap*. Let me see Thomas Edison turning the light on. Transport me to the moment when Van Leeuwenhoek peered, for the first time, into the life of a single cell. Most of all, I want to sit in the audience at the premiere of *The Rite of Spring*, a ballet composed by Igor Stravinsky. I want to be in the audience not only because I love *The Rite of Spring* and am intrigued by its rhythm, but because there was a drama taking place in that concert hall—a drama that had to do with rhythm, and with the human heart, and with human nature—and I just love dramas, especially if I don't have to stay until it's all over.

Igor Stravinsky and I have a common past. No, we have never met. But I was listening to him. To his music, I mean. It started during my military service. I joined the army at 18. After a convoluted path that included a rigorous boot-camp and about a month in the Transportation and Logistic Service to which I was assigned by a miserable clerical mistake, I was eventually stationed in a military base in the center of Tel Aviv. About the nature of my main mission there I can divulge absolutely nothing (top secret, you know). But this I can say: at the beginning of my service there, I was assigned to gate-guard duty.

I was assigned to the South Gate of the base, once a week, for two nightly shifts of two hours each. The guard-booth was small. It was raining non-stop, and it was cold. I wore a heavy coat, with an Uzzi sub-machine gun strapped over my shoulder. It was boring and endless.

The South Gate was very close to a large hospital that specialized in delivering babies. And as mothers were laboring and babies were delivered, the cries of agony penetrated my mind with increasing frequency.

'This can't go on,' I thought, and for the next shift I came equipped. I inserted a Walkman into an inside pocket of my jacket and ran the wire—with a single ear-bud at its end—underneath my coat and all the way to my ear. I zipped up my coat and placed the hood over my head. This solution, I thought, would be ideal—nobody could see me listening to music, which was prohibited during guard duty, and I could fight boredom with art.

Things turned out differently. The only cassette I could find was Igor Stravinsky's *The Rite of Spring*. And so, I played it over and over. *The Rite of Spring* (an orchestral piece but also a ballet) opens with themes of primitive rituals celebrating the beginning of spring. It ends with the sacrifice of a young girl who dances herself to death. If the subject matter sounds lovely, its interpretation is even more unsettling. And most noticeably because of the irregular rhythm of the composition. It isn't the 1-2-3, 1-2-3, 1-2-3, rhythm of a waltz, nor is it the more common 1-2-3-4, 1-2-3-4 in most popular songs. To create The Rite, the legend goes, Stravinsky wrote the combination 1-2 on some pieces of paper and 1-2-3 on others; he threw these notes into the air and let them land on the floor of his studio. He then randomly picked up the notes from the floor and let this random non-orderly order dictate the rhythm of The Rite. The final result is enigmatic, primitive, passionate, powerful, and, in terms of rhythm, irregularly-irregular.

I wish I could have been there, at the Théatre des Champs-Elysées in Paris on the night of May 29, 1913, at *The Rite of Spring* premiere. The house was full to the brim with dignitaries, art lovers, and artists, corridors and stairways included. As *The Rite* began, the audience responded with initial unease; then there was a terrific uproar. It turned into a riot. Carl Van Vechten, a journalist, reported that the man behind him started to "beat rhythmically on top of my head with his fists." A member of the orchestra reported that "everything available was tossed in our direction, but we continued to play on."

What caused the riot, nobody knows. It might have been the primal, violent music, or the wild dancing. Perhaps it was all staged as a publicity stunt. I wish I could have been there, at the theater, to confirm my own theory: 'It's the irregularly-irregular rhythm, stupid! It's about the rhythm of the heart.'

Imagine a world in which Stravinsky's rhythm rules: no more predictable rhythms—no nights, mornings, afternoons; no summer, fall, winter, or spring; no breakfast, lunch, or dinner; no church bells tolling. Now imagine even worse—that you suddenly become acutely aware that your heartbeat has lost its regularity. Instead of order, disorder! And sense of danger. And the fear of impending death.

2.

On an autumn Sunday, just after his morning coffee, 57 year old Adam Bloom became aware of his own heartbeat. It wasn't the rapid heart rate he remembered from his youth, the kind he would experience after a three mile run, or when he fell in love at first sight. Nor was it the slower, relaxed heartbeat he sometimes noticed after a class of deep-breathing meditation at the YMCA. It was an ominous rhythm, unpredictable and irregular. A heartbeat so chaotic, he would tell himself later, that for a long time he lost his faith in world order.

In an essay he wrote in a biology class in high school, Adam, a man who would years later become a mechanical engineer, wrote: "my heart is no more than a simple pump." He calculated that with a normal heart rate and a normal life span (78.6 years), a heart would have to beat

2,891,851,200 times! "A durable, long-lasting pump," he wrote, "but a mere pump nevertheless." His teacher advised him to revise his essay.

In the revised version of his essay, Adam wrote: "To many, the heart is a mystery. Some romantic souls see it as the seat of human emotions (perhaps because their heart races at the sight of a loved one); others consider it a mere mechanical pump. The truth lies in between these two views: the heart is a sophisticated pump which adapts to the needs of the body by adjusting its rate and contractility. That's it."

Adam then added: "Even the mystery of the origin of the heartbeat is not a mystery anymore. In 1906, Martin Flack, a medical student who worked under the supervision of Arthur Keith, solved the 'mystery.'" Arthur and his wife were bicycling through the beautiful cherry orchards near their cottage in Kent, England. Upon their return, Martin announced with great excitement that as he was studying the heart of a mole under the microscope, he discovered a wonderful structure, a group of cells in the atrium (the upper chamber) of the heart. This group of cells, Flack and Keith believed, was the long-sought-after site of origin of the heartbeat—the pacemaker. From the pacemaker, the electrical current propagates, in an orderly wave, through the entire heart. And this, in turn, results in a coordinated contraction." In Adam's mind, it all became as clear as the sky on a cloudless day: the heart is a pump controlled by its own electrical system. It holds no secrets.

Years later, in the emergency department, Dr. Gold told Adam, "Your heart is misbehaving. It is beating faster than it should, and its rhythm is irregular. We call it 'atrial fibrillation.'"

"The normal rhythm generated in your pacemaker is overwhelmed by rapid, irregular electrical discharges that originate elsewhere—in the tissues around the pacemaker. As a result, your atrium, the upper chamber of your heart, quivers. Instead of coordinated contraction, instead of regular rhythm," the doctor said, "we are dealing with an irregular rhythm and an uncoordinated contraction."

Dr. Gold explained the treatment options: "we will start with medications to control the heart rate and restore its normal rhythm. If these measures fail, we will perform cardio-version using electrical shock. It is as if we turned off your heart for a moment and pressed the re-start button."

That didn't appeal to Adam, but when Dr. Gold described the many symptoms and complications that would ensue should Adam decide to forgo treatment—shortness of breath, light-headedness, loss of consciousness, swelling of the legs, and even, God forbid, a stroke—Adam understood the severity of his situation.

After several attempts, Adam's heart returned to a normal rhythm. He gained new insight into the wonders of his heart and the universe around it.

'How could I truly understand the mechanism of the heart, any heart, my heart?' This question was natural to Adam, for he was, after all, an engineer. He answered such questions with self-assured certainty: in order to design a perfect skyscraper, he would observe the collapse of poorly-designed buildings; to fully understand flight, he would watch airplanes nose-dive into the ground. After his own heart had lost its normal rhythm, Adam found comfort in the realization that this failure was the key to understanding the wondrous design of his heart.

3.

My interest in the jumping spider stems only from my wish to find the source of my own heart's rhythm. And yet, I can't ignore the little spider's charisma, its charm, its romantic nature. It is small—about the size of a pencil eraser—and hairy. It wears its crunchy skeleton on the outside, like the armor of a medieval knight. It has eight legs, and it walks slowly, but it jumps with the agility of an Olympic athlete. To attract its female counterpart, the male spider will display its hairs, show off its more colorful parts, dance in a zig-zag movement, and make buzzing and drum-roll sounds. Who could resist such a song-and-dance show of affection?

A long time ago, the jumping spider abandoned its net-knitting. It had no time for elaborate net construction and no patience to sit idly and wait for its prey to be caught in its net. Instead, it began to actively hunt its prey by jumping at it. First, it needed to identify its prey. Like a cat, it would stealthily stalk and then pounce. It would do so using its eight eyes, which allow for a high-resolution, almost 360-degree, panoramic view of the environment.

In a laboratory at Cornell University, scientists working with Professor Ronald R. Hoy were able to gently introduce a miniature, hair-sized electrode into the brain of several jumping spiders. They measured the electrical activity in the spiders' brains in response to images projected on a screen in front of them: images of a fly (a prey) and of other jumping spiders (potential mating partners or competitors). The researchers then repeated the experiments while covering different sets of the spiders' eyes. The results were astonishing: put an image of a fly in front of a jumping spider and its brain would fire as vividly as a seismograph during an earthquake; cover even one set of eyes and the electrical activity in the spider's brain would die down. The jumping spider doesn't just see its prey; it is able to integrate and compute stimuli from four different pairs of eyes into one coherent message: 'This is my prey!' Or, 'This is my mate! Whatever it is, I recognize it!' The spider must possess at least some form of cognition.

In a different set of experiments, the same group of researchers were able to prove, two years later, that the jumping spider cannot only see and recognize its prey, it can also hear at a distance of up to 3 meters. The spider's brain, mind you, is no bigger than a poppy seed.

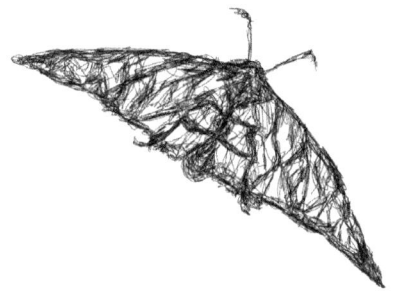

If the jumping spider doesn't fill your heart with awe (do you belong to AA—arachnophobe anonymous?), perhaps you would be more impressed by the mystery of the Monarch butterfly migration. The Monarch is a lovely creature whose body is light and beautifully painted in yellow-orange to match the sunshine, whose wings are as thin and semi-translucent as onion skin—an embodiment of air and light. Every autumn, millions of Monarch butterflies migrate from the ominous, freezing territories of North America to Mexico and Florida. Scientists claim that the Monarchs orient themselves by using a highly-specialized circadian clock integrated with a sun-compass located in their antennas. There are several theories attempting to explain the Monarch's ability to migrate with elegance and precision, and no theory is accepted by all, a sign that the jury is still out. With a brain made of a few cells, the Monarch can find its way—a distance of 3,000 miles—better than I can find my way to the post office in a neighboring town, even with my GPS turned on.

How can the jumping spider, whose brain is no bigger than a poppy seed, perceive and analyze signals of light and sound? How can it detect its small, moving prey, compute the distance to its prey, calculate the forces it should use for jumping? And how can the Monarch butterfly, with a brain even smaller, find its course? I wonder: what is the driving force behind the spider's behaviors—the drive to hunt and to mate? Does it feel hunger? Is the Monarch butterfly a romantic? Perhaps even self-aware? And what is the force that compels the Monarch butterfly to seek new territories?

4.

Suppose you stumble upon a revolutionary idea. I am talking about a big idea. Perhaps you think the Earth is round while everyone else still thinks it's flat. Perhaps you believe the sun is at the center of the universe, not the Earth. Your idea might intrigue some, but upset almost everyone else. How far would you go in sticking to your idea, defending it, fighting for it? What if you have absolute confidence in your idea? What if you stumbled upon what you believe is The Theory of Everything?

Baruch Spinoza, a 17th century philosopher, came upon such big ideas. Rebecca Goldstein, a philosopher and novelist, called Spinoza the "renegade Jew" who gave us modernity. Antonio Damasio, a professor of neuroscience at the University of Southern California, found inspiration in Spinoza's ideas for his own understanding of consciousness. Albert Einstein found his own God in

Spinoza's: "I believe in Spinoza's God," Einstein wrote, "who reveals himself in the lawful harmony of the world, not in a God who concerns himself with the fate and the doings of mankind." And Joaquin Garcia, a Spanish man and a civil servant, skipped work for 6 years, just so he could study Spinoza (and no one at work noticed).

Baruch Spinoza was born into a world of intolerance. In 1492, his ancestors, Jews of Sephardic descent, were expelled from Spain and fled to Portugal. They then fled the Portuguese inquisition for fear of forced religious conversion and execution. They finally arrived in the Netherlands, a more tolerant land, where they were allowed to practice Judaism.

Intolerance was not directed only toward other religions, but toward new ideas in general. Galileo Galilei, for example, insisted that the sun, not the Earth, lies motionless at the center of the universe. The inquisition, in return, found him "vehemently suspect of heresy." He was placed under house arrest for the rest of his life, and publication of any of his work was forbidden (Italy, 1633).

Intolerance was not limited to the Christian world. In Amsterdam, Uriel da Costa, a philosopher and a skeptic from Portugal, was called before the rabbinic leadership for uttering blasphemous views against Judaism. He was fined a large sum of money and excommunicated. Years later, in front of the whole congregation, in a crowded synagogue, Uriel da Costa read from a written confession detailing his numerous transgressions. Then, leaning against a column, his hands tied, his back bare, he was publicly given 39 lashings (the maximum allowed was 40). He was then forced to lie on the floor while the entire congregation trampled over him. Only then did the Rabbi announce da Costa's excommunication to be lifted. In 1640, demoralized and depressed, da Costa shot himself in the head. The first bullet missed the target; the second did him in.

Spinoza's ideas about the nature of man and God were radical. Synagogue officials warned Spinoza, then offered him a large bribe to recant his ideas. A fellow Jew attempted to stab Spinoza on the steps of the synagogue. Protected by a large cloak, the knife barely missed Spinoza's slim body. Spinoza kept the torn cloak as a souvenir, for years.

In July, 1656, the Jewish congregation of Amsterdam issued a writ of *cherem* (excommunication, expulsion from the community) against the 23-year-old Spinoza. The document does not detail the transgressions Spinoza was accused of, but his views must have been more abominable than da Costa's, and his persistence more intolerable, for unlike da Costa before him, Spinoza's excommunication was never lifted. Even for a time of great intolerance, the language of the writ stands out as being unusually harsh: "Cursed be he [Spinoza] by day and cursed be he by night; cursed be he when he lies down, and cursed be he when he rises up; cursed be he when he goes out, and cursed be he when he comes in… The anger and wrath of the Lord will rage against this man…"

Born into a community of exiles—Jews who fled their country because they believed in a different God—Spinoza became an exile within his own community for believing in a different idea of God.

"This compels me," Spinoza said about the writ of excommunication, "to nothing that I should not otherwise have done."

Spinoza withdrew to a life of solitude. In a humble study room, he systematically formulated a deep philosophical view of the whole universe.

The beat of my heart; the jump of a spider; the migration of a butterfly—where are all these drawing their signal from? Could Spinoza's "Theory of Everything" resolve the mystery better than contemporary scientists?

5.

My father told me that when he was a little child he used to imagine that the voices coming from his radio were of people living inside it. Tiny news announcers, little singers, and miniature music band members would share the little space, taking turns to recite the news, sing and play classical music. "I turned the dial as fast as I could," he told me, "and imagined a burst of activity taking place: the news announcer was told to quickly quiet down, and the band had to rush into their positions at the microphone, the drums, the trumpets, and start playing. So much chaos took place in my imagination as I turned the dial, that it made me laugh," he said.

When I heard my father's radio story—I was myself a kid at the time—my own imagination ignited: I saw little people crossing from the electrical socket and through the wires into the TV set that stood in our living room. These people—news anchors, actors, and musicians—sat quietly in a dark corner inside the TV box, wearing an expression of great anticipation. And when their turn would come, they would take the main stage, and their image would be projected on the screen for us to see. At night, when the TV was off, they would return through the wires to their homes.

The other day, I typed "Baruch Spinoza" into the Google search bar. I wanted to know more about the life of the 17th century Dutch philosopher and about his ideas. And in the tradition of imaginative people, I wanted to imagine an immense, dark library residing within my laptop with busy librarians swinging into action, searching for answers in heavy books that smell of wood. Instead, I realized that this was getting harder and harder for me to imagine—my laptop is too thin to hold even the smallest of miniature libraries. And it is wireless; even the skinniest of librarians couldn't walk in through the electrical cord, and nobody could leave when I turn off the power.

And still, as I typed, as I tapped into Google's tree of knowledge, an ocean of information presented itself: Spinoza did not conduct even one experiment to test his ideas. He didn't observe nature to understand nature. His was a pure thought-experiment. A theory. In an orderly, mathematical fashion, one proposal led to another until he reached what he thought was an indisputable conclusion.

In Spinoza's world, the words 'God' and 'Nature' are used interchangeably. God is Nature and Nature is God. And Nature is infinite and at the same time a single substance. You and everything you see and experience is a single substance of the universe. You and everything around you are just different "attributes" of the same thing: Nature. In Spinoza's words: "By God, I mean a being absolutely infinite, that is to say, a substance consisting of infinite attributes, each of which expresses eternal and infinite essence."

Here is how I understand Spinoza's theory. In my father's imagination, people were separate from each other and from the radio box within which they resided. They spoke to him, and he listened. He turned the dial, and they had to quickly adjust. All things were separate and acted upon each other. In my childhood imagination, people needed to squeeze themselves through wires in orders to reach the TV set. In today's world, though, there are no wires, and I enter a universe of wisdom by clicking on a keyboard.

Spinoza, I thought, just took this sequence of ideas a step further. In his world, there is no need for wires, nor for a wireless relationship among things. Instead, we are all made of one substance called Nature. There is no cause and effect. There is no way to modify current existence or change consequences. It is all predetermined and one—a universe in its purest form of infinite freedom.

Spinoza's Theory of Everything is foreign to my daily experience. I just know that I have come to this world and will exit it; that I occupy a physical space; that I have an effect on inanimate objects and living creatures; that I love people that are separate from me.

And yet, there is a great temptation in thinking that I am just a part of Nature, one with God, inseparable from the Universe. After all, If I could believe in Spinoza's philosophy, I would free myself from the need to answer how the jumping spider finds its prey, the migrating butterfly its destination, and my heart its own rhythm. These need no outside signal anymore. And everything is just an attribute of Nature.

ASLEEP

The stars peacefully land
on your body,
a blanket of lights
in the darkest
of nights.

The feathers calmly lift
your head,
a pillow of sights
in the coldest
of nights.

Asleep,
you gather the dreams
of the people who lived—
a storm of lightning, thunder,
and the morning's scent of wet grass.

RELATIONSHIPS

CARDIOLOGY OF THE BUMBLEBEE

I am a bumblebee.
My weightless wings flutter,
but my heart
is heavy as a rock,
rolling down a mountain.

On my way to taste
your nectar,
I am buzzing,
but my soul rumbles,
and my heart is an ocean of tears.

Where are you, my love?
And where will your heart be?
Will your love for me last?
Or will you shed me like an old coat,
shake me off like a snake's skin?

I will fly to you, love,
bubbling with lust.
I will ride the winds
along rays of early sunshine.
I will glitter your face with
morning's dew.

When I return to my hive,
I will tell my Queen
that your love for me lives
in my wings that flutter
like a heart
before it stops.

LOVE BY THE NUMBERS

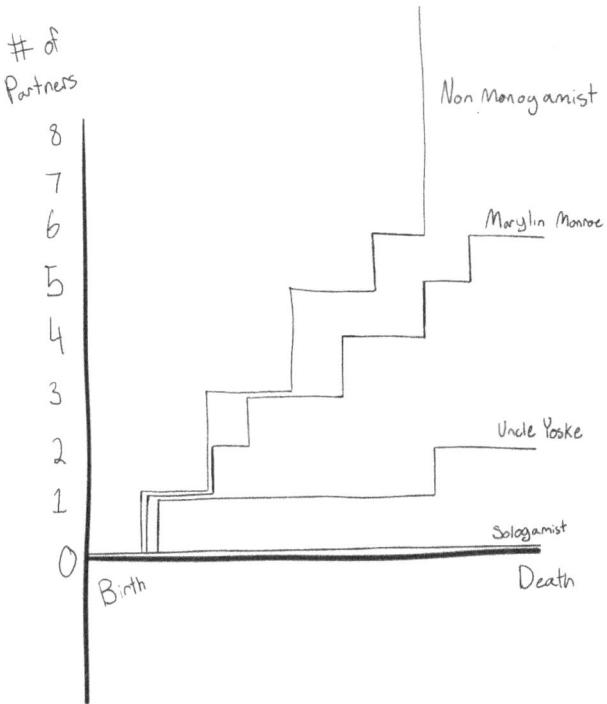

N=1

The spectrum of human romantic relationships seems more confusing than ever. Monogamy is still as simple as plain vanilla, but when exactly do you start calling someone a serial monogamist? What is the difference between serial monogamy and polygamy? What the heck is "sologamy"? And what is the difference between plain old cheating and polyamory?

With these questions on my mind, I decided to clear things up, at least for myself, and write down a few very short stories. The first is about my uncle Yoske who, in my imagination, comes as close as one could ever be to a monogamist.

My first memory of Yoske—I was about 5 or 7 at the time—is from a wedding, or perhaps it was a funeral, I am not sure. He was a short, stout man with a few hairs on his head and thick glasses in a black frame. One of his eyelids, I think it was the left one, drooped. At first, I thought Yoske was winking at me, but his face was serious. I saw him pacing back and forth, away from the crowd of guests, contemplating something of great consequence. He was whistling to himself an unfamiliar and repetitive tune, composed of only a few notes.

"Let's say hi to uncle Yoske," my mom said. She took me by the hand and walked with me toward Yoske. He stopped whistling and stood still for a moment, smiled only slightly, and when I extended my arm to shake his hand, he said, "Sorry, young man, I don't shake hands. You know, there are billions of bugs out there; we don't want to help them spread around, do we?

Over the next several years, I learned more about Yoske. He had emigrated to Israel from Poland and had become a successful entrepreneur. He owned and operated an aluminum factory in downtown Haifa. In a series of transactions with several partners, he made a small, yet significant fortune. My father, a businessman himself, told me to never become a partner of uncle Yoske. "Yoske will come up with an idea," my father warned me, "and ask you to invest your hard-earned money. In the end, you will be left with his worthless idea, while he would run away with your money." I took notes. I was about 10 at the time. I wanted to be either an artist or a pilot. I never intended to engage in the unforgiving world of aluminum.

There are good-intention-Yoske stories too. One year, during Hanukkah, Yoske gave me an aluminum *dreidel* he had made in his factory. Like all dreidels, Yoske's dreidel was a four-sided spin-top with one Hebrew letter etched onto each of the sides. Together, these letters formed an acronym for the phrase 'Great Miracle Happened There.' The dreidel brought excitement to my heart. I immediately saw myself playing the Dreidel Game. Yoske's dreidel, though, did not collaborate. It spun awkwardly, defied the laws of physics, and, perhaps miraculously, it always fell with the side showing M, for Miracle, up.

My mom admired Yoske. "My sister, Hannah, is the luckiest woman on Earth," my mom used to say. "She married Yoske, a man as solid as a rock. A man solely dedicated to his wife. A family man." Indeed, Yoske was married to my aunt Hannah until death set them apart. Together, they raised two beautiful girls. Yoske had no interest in other women. Each morning, Hannah would greet Yoske at their kitchen table with a glass of milk and two butter cookies she had baked according to a recipe that she invented. At lunchtime, he would return from the factory so that they could eat lunch together. And at nights, they watched *Mabat*, the daily TV news show, then went to bed. The couple's life was monotonous, without undue drama, and, from the outside, happy.

When the couple was in their 80s, auntie Hannah became pleasantly confused. Doctors said it was Alzheimer's disease. One day, she left the house. A policeman brought her back after several hours. Days later, she died.

One or two years after aunt Hannah passed, Uncle Yoske met Ruth. Ruth took one look at Hannah's cookie recipe and said that she could make these butter cookies, no problem. When Yoske tasted Ruth's cookies, he nodded his head in approval. The new couple married a few months later.

N>1 (IN SEQUENCE, SOMETIMES RAPID)

Like my uncle Yoske who was *almost* a perfect monogamist, Elizabeth Taylor was *almost* a true serial-monogamist. After all, she had, at times, romantic relationships with more than one man. I could have searched further, but these true serial-monogamists are not easy to come by, and their lives are not even half as interesting as Taylor's. Therefore, I present to you: Liz.

Elizabeth Taylor was born a star. Shortly thereafter, she

became a child prodigy. Then, an adult Hollywood star. As a doctor, I observed that the process wasn't devoid of life-threatening complications: During the shooting of *National Velvet* (1944), Liz fell from a horse and hurt her back; years later, in *A Place in the Sun* (1951), in the famous fainting scene, Liz, then a delicate, fragile 19-year-old, dramatically collapsed. She did it so convincingly that, watching the scene, I felt a sudden urge to jump into the screen and resuscitate her. It turned out she was just acting; and in the 1960s, while performing as the ruler of the Kingdom of Egypt in *Cleopatra* (finally released in 1963), Liz caught pneumonia (the story of *Cleopatra* takes place in sunny, hot Egypt, but the film was initially shot in England, where the cold weather was blamed for Liz's medical near-catastrophe). She was hospitalized, had a tracheotomy, and almost died. Hollywood, I am telling you, is risky business.

Liz was so beautiful that she could steal the heart of a man like a master thief in a midday robbery. Her face was perfectly symmetric, her smile inviting. Her eyes were like a picture, framed by a double row of eyelashes (doctors call it *distichiasis*—the result of a rare genetic mutation at the FOXC2 gene).

How much of a serial-monogamist was Taylor? Well, she was married eight times, but to only seven men. Puzzled? The answer is simple: Taylor married Richard Burton twice (and also divorced him twice).

To prevent further confusion, I have summarized Taylor's relationships in what follows:

Conrad Hilton Junior (married, 1950; divorced, 1951): yes, that Hilton—the son of the founder of Hilton Hotels and hence a man of means. Also known as the uncle of Paris Hilton. He was a gambler, a drinker, and a womanizer. Not the best marriage material.

Michael Wilding (married, 1952; divorced, 1957): An artist and an actor who was 20 years older than Taylor. Taylor and Wilding had two children. He was never the most popular star in Britain, but came close, in 1949, as the second most popular. He was married 4 times. He also had a short romance with Marie McDonald, an actress who answered to the name The Body.

Mike Todd (married, 1957): A film and theater producer who won the Academy Award for Best Picture for *Around the World in 80 Days*. He was 23 years older than Taylor and the only husband Taylor did not divorce. They had a daughter together. Their relationship was described as tempestuous. He died in a private plane accident in 1958.

Eddie Fisher (Married, 1959; divorced 1964): A singer and actor who sold millions of records and hosted his own TV show. He had an affair with Taylor while being married to Taylor's best friend, Debbie Reynolds. Oh, Taylor—what a home wrecker! What a scandal!

Richard Burton (Married, 1964; divorced, 1974; married again, 1975; divorced again, 1976): Burton, an actor famous for pretending to be (rather than not to be) Hamlet—a man nominated for an Academy Award seven times, never to win an Oscar—was still one of the best paid actors ever. In a biography by Melvin Bragg, *Richard Burton, A Life*, Burton said about his first impression of Taylor: "She was so extraordinarily beautiful ... She was undeniably gorgeous ... She was, in short, too bloody much, and not only that, she was totally ignoring me." Their affair was a global scandal, relentlessly covered by the media, for at the time they met, on the movie set of *Cleopatra*, they were both married—to other people. The Vatican condemned the couple for their "erotic vagrancy." Later, Taylor reminisced about her relationship with Burton: "It was fun and it was dark—oceans of tears, but some good times too." To lighten the darkness, to stop her tears, Burton gave Taylor the Taylor-Burton Diamond he bought for $1,050,000. She said, "Big girls need big diamonds."

Then came John Warner, a senator from Virginia (m.1976; div. 1982) and Larry Fortensky, a construction worker known only as Taylor's last husband (1991-1996).

I would tell you more, but I think that you get the idea. Taylor was a woman who loved to fall in love and to be passionately loved, but for her, staying in love, for long, was just an impossible mission.

Was Taylor's love life happier, more fulfilling, than my uncle Yoske's almost perfectly monogamous life? She described her multiple affairs not as a choice, but as fate: "I've always admitted that I'm ruled by my passions," she admitted, and on another occasion, she said: "I am a very committed wife. And I should be committed too—for being married so many times."

N>1 (ALL TOGETHER NOW)

A patient of mine, George, told me that he was starting to feel the seven-year itch. He wondered if he should start seeing other women besides his wife.

"I am just a urologist," I told him, "not a priest, not a marriage counselor." And then I added, as if to myself, "once the ship has left the safe harbor of monogamy and sailed into the vast ocean of non-monogamous relationships, it encounters stormy, turbulent waters."

Later, at home, I searched the scientific literature for guidance.

I should, I told myself, start with definitions. While the pure monogamist has one life-long partner, and the serial-monogamist has one partner at a time, the non-monogamist indulges in two or more simultaneous relationships over a period of time. To borrow from the gastronomy world, the non-monogamist might say, "It is true that my partner is a wonderful cook, but does that necessarily mean I should never try a different cook at another restaurant?"

I then categorized non-monogamous relationships, and the best way to start, it seemed, was by asking the question: are you trying to keep the other relationship secret? If you keep your other relationship secret, if you hide its existence—you are a cheater. And once the cheating is revealed, guilty carnal pleasures and shared whispered secrets typically turn into a painful, shameful drama. If you are a celebrity, the exposure might turn into a scandal. Your primary relationship may end and so might your relationship with your cheating partner. Playing the numbers game, you may find yourself going, at a blink of an eye, from two or more relationships to none.

Matters turn even more interesting if you and your partner agree to a non-monogamous relationship. Researchers, such as Dr. Terri D. Conley from the Department of Psychology at the University of Michigan, call these types of arrangements consensually non-monogamous relationships. Researchers estimate that 3.5-5% of individuals in a relationship are consensually non-monogamous. But is consensual non-monogamy satisfying? And is it of high quality? In one investigation, published in the journal *Perspectives in Psychological Science*, Conley tried to address these questions.

Conley further divided consensual non-monogamy into three distinct groups: the swingers, the polyamorous, and those who partake in an open relationship (to which my grandma would say, "So open minded that the brain is coming out").

The swingers, according to Conley, engage in sexual relationships with partners other than their primary partner. They do so at parties and other social events arranged for that matter. The relationships outside of their primary relationship are sexual and are not intended to be romantic or long-term. Polyamorous couples, on the other hand, say "the-more-love-the-merrier"—they agree to have close, emotional, romantic, and sexual relationships with partners outside of their primary relationships. And last, couples who practice an open relationship allow each other to participate in sexual relationships outside of their own as long as long-term romantic or emotional relationships are avoided. They engage in their other relationships separately and do not typically discuss the dates they have outside their primary relationship.

Conley recruited most of the participants to her study online through websites devoted to non-monogamous relationships and through the volunteer section of craigslist.com. A minority of participants (12%) were psychology undergraduate students who received credit for their participation in the study. Altogether, Conley evaluated 1507 individuals in monogamous relationships and 617 individuals in non-monogamous relationships. This sample was large enough to draw conclusions about the differences between monogamous and non-monogamous relationships.

Conley asked the participants about their satisfaction with their relationships and about their trust in their partners. She also measured the participants' sexual jealousy, passionate love, and commitment. She did so using questionnaires that had been specifically designed and were found reliable for research purposes.

The results were astonishing. According to prior studies, lay-people believe that monogamous relationships are more trusting, committed, passionate, and sexually satisfying. Monogamy, the lay-people believed, is also less likely to involve jealousy. Dr. Conley's study showed that the two groups—monogamous and non-monogamous—reported a similar degree of satisfaction in their relationships, in their commitment to each other, and in their levels of passionate love. Moreover, non-monogamous participants reported more trust and less jealousy in their relationships.

Should George, my seven-year itch patient, turn non-monogamous? Shouldn't we all?

Reading Dr. Conley's article, I was almost ready to jump off the sofa, perhaps even jump on the sofa, in an enthusiastic *aha* moment. I wanted to run out the door and spread the news. I wanted to come to you all—my neighbors in Marquette and the Upper Peninsula, and people in general, wherever you are—with a strong recommendation: to quickly abandon monogamy.

Then I started thinking. I came up with two main arguments against the conclusions of Dr. Conley's study. First, the participants in the study were either undergraduate students of psychology, or volunteers recruited through Craigslist. I assumed that undergraduate psychology students and those using Craigslist—searching for a gently used coffee table, or raving, in the Rants and Raves section of Craigslist, about a loophole in the Ice Bucket Challenge—may not be the best sample of the entire population.

Once the second argument formed in my mind, I just had to contact Dr. Conley herself. "Your study," I wrote to her in an e-mail, "seems to provide a snapshot in time, but is there any study that examines the long-term satisfaction/happiness in the relationships of couples in a consensual non-monogamous relationship? And what effect do non-monogamous relationships have on measures such as financial stability of the family and on the ability of such families to raise happy, successful children?"

Dr. Conley was kind. She e-mailed me back the next morning. "There are as of yet no longitudinal studies of polyamorous/CNM [consensual non-monogamous] relationships. There is very little interest in funding this topic, although I personally find it fascinating!"

Lacking any scientific research comparing the long-term effects of monogamous and non-monogamous relationships, we are left with only anecdotal evidence in the form of stories told by individuals and couples. In her letter, Dr. Conley referred me to her colleague, Elisabeth Sheff, a sociologist whose approach was different than that of Dr. Conley's. In her book 'Stories from the Polycule', she did not seek to compare individuals in monogamous and non-monogamous relationships. Instead, she sought to document the experiences of polyamorists. She asked polyamorists to tell her their life stories. The book is an anthology, a collection of such stories.

In an interview by Thorntree Press published on YouTube, Sheff admitted that it was hard for her to track down past polyamorists whose relationships ended painfully, but she did compile enough stories to paint a vivid picture of polyamorous relationships. Several stories describe the formation of polyamorous relationships. Some chose polyamory intentionally, while others just fell into it, finding themselves in love with more than one person. These individuals then had to add an additional "puzzle-piece" person into their primary existing relationship. The extra piece, Sheff says, doesn't always fit in.

Other stories in Sheff's book shed light on how a poly-family functions, as in "what it is like to come back home to more than one partner?" Another section in the book tells the stories of kids in poly-families and yet another section describes very long-term polyamory relationships. In the end, Sheff says, some polyamory relationships continue to exist for a long period of time, sometimes taking the form of non-romantic, non-sexual relationships.

As in stories about monogamous relationships, the end isn't always happy. Sheff doesn't hesitate to tell her own Full Circle story: her initial attempt at polyamory, she tells the interviewer, was "ill-fated, poorly-conceived, badly-executed, and all-around disastrous—it turned out badly." Later, she had fallen in love and married the woman who is still her wife. When the opportunity presented itself, and she met yet another lovable woman, Sheff considered polyamory again, but her partner expressed concerns. Having experienced a painful polyamorous relationship in the past, Sheff decided she didn't want to be in a relationship with two people who didn't want to share her. She decided not to pursue a romantic relationship with the other woman. And later, she found herself happy with the stability of her monogamous marriage.

Can we learn anything from the stories others—whether in monogamous or non-monogamous relationships—tell us? Can the results of even the best of studies inform us as to which type of relationship to pursue? Isn't it simpler to abandon relationships altogether, choose sologamy, and marry yourself?

N=0 (I'M THE SPECIAL AND ONLY 1)

Are you tired of looking for Mr. or Ms. Right? Being alone no longer means being lonely. An increasing number of women (and a few men too) abandon loneliness. Instead, they choose solitude. To celebrate the occasion, they marry themselves. And marrying yourself has a name now—it is called 'sologamy.'

What a celebration sologamy is. A celebration of freedom, independence, self-respect, and, most of all, self-love. But also a celebration similar to that practiced in a traditional relationship. First, you have to propose. You should be dramatic—kneel down and ask yourself, "Will you marry me?" Then, you have to accept, and why wouldn't you? After all, you love yourself and are destined to live with yourself for the rest of your life. Besides, would you propose in the first place if you knew you would refuse? An engagement ring follows. A guest list.

Wedding invitations. A wedding cake. A photographer. A band. A master of ceremonies. You get the idea: It's like a wedding. No — It is a wedding.

Japanese women are especially sologamy-enthusiastic. News From Elsewhere, on BBC.com, reports that a travel agency in Kyoto, Japan is offering a two-day "solo-wedding" package that includes "choosing your own special gown, bouquet and hairstyle, a limousine service, a stay at a hotel and a commemorative photo album."

Grace Gelder, a London-based portrait photographer, also found the right person she knew all her life—herself. According to The Guardian, Gelder's parents were open-minded about the idea, and her grandma said: "Oh, you always think of something new, Grace." Some acquaintances felt that the idea was a bit narcissistic. She proposed to herself while sitting on a park bench on Parliament Hill. She decided a wedding ceremony will make the agreement with herself stick. At the ceremony, Gelder says, "I was met by what felt like a sea of beaming faces." Her sister was the only family member who attended, although Gelder's mother and father sent supportive text messages. There was a ring, a vintage wedding dress, and a close friend who served as a celebrant. In a picture taken at the event, I saw a crowd of young people waving a sea of hands, extending their arms toward Gelder in an expression of happiness and love, their faces lit with wide smiles.

Is Gelder's sologamy a commitment for life? "And just because I married myself," Grace Gelder said, "it doesn't mean that I'm not open to the idea of sharing a wedding with someone else one day." On her website, Grace Gelder quotes Oscar Wilde: "To love oneself is the beginning of a lifelong romance."

As I approach the end of this series of chapters, the time has come for reflection.

Isn't a relationship, I ask myself, any relationship, merely a solution to a problem? To stay alone is lonesome, and for the problem of loneliness, the social script prescribes a relationship. "Take monogamy, twice a day," I hear an imaginary doctor tell a patient. One in the morning before you go to work and one in the evening when you come back home, and never stop, for the rest of your life." But monogamy, which looks, at the beginning, like a good solution to an existential problem, may create other problems: even if taken with a spoonful of sugar, monogamy doesn't work for everyone, and side effects may include: boredom, dissatisfaction, disappointment, self-pity, and bursts of anger. Some users may experience feelings of being ignored, even unloved. Others sit in the corner and cry.

Searching for a solution to the side effects of monogamy, some lonely hearts stumble upon a relationship with another person, or persons. This comes with initial elation, a sense of adventure and discovery, and it may even satisfy carnal and emotional needs, but if the new relationship is kept a secret, a consuming guilt may develop on one side and a sense of betrayal on the other; and if the information is shared (or discovered), anger and pain will typically ensue. A seemingly good solution creates a new problem. And the solution to the new problem? Yet another relationship?

In my mind, I see sailors in search of an island of love. I ask myself: isn't love a particular story we are persuaded to believe in—a princess in the tall tower waiting for her rescue; a princess kissing a frog; a happily-ever-after life? But in the real world, each sailor navigates their own course, conducts their own experiment at sea. 'Sail along the river,' the sailors are told, 'and don't stray.' But she meets waves, high and ominous. He draws into deep, turbulent water. On their way down the river, mysterious blue caves along the shore will seem inviting, and narrow, serpentine tributaries will whisper for them to come and taste the water. With each turn of the plot—a discovery of self and other—the sailors will draw closer to safe land and find a cure for their loneliness. Or not.

FOLIE-A-DEUX

Angelina was seeking a companion. She responded to a personal ad in a single's magazine. She was 23, Angelo was 27, love bloomed, and within a week the couple got married.

At age 8, Angelo was diagnosed with paranoid schizophrenia. He had delusions and hallucinations. He was often visited by three "demons," imaginary figures he named Romanoff, The Baron, and LaBelle.

On their wedding night, Angelina saw Angelo become possessed by Romanoff. Angelo told Angelina that he was the god of the ocean, and that he had known her throughout her childhood. She was initially scared, but over the next two years, when Angelo was visited by Romanoff and his other demons at increasing frequency, she became accustomed to Angelo's delusions and integrated them into her own world.

In the world they had built, there was Romanoff, "the fallen angel with greyish-black wings" who held "a sword with gems upon it." There was LaBelle, the "tall beautiful lady dressed in silver with long silver hair ... who carried a chalice full of blood" drawn from Angelo's enemies. And there was The Baron, a tall gentlemen dressed in black who carried a sword.

Angelina and Angelo were socially isolated. They experienced financial difficulties. They had to move from one state to another in search of a steady job for Angelo.

The couple continued to hear voices. Romanoff, for example, told them that Angelo would soon die and Angelina would be raped.

The couple bought a gun.

One night, while dining in a restaurant, Angelo saw two strangers laughing. He thought they were laughing at him. Angelina and Angelo left the restaurant and returned to their home, where Angelo was once again possessed by Romanoff. "The enemies were laughing at us. You must kill them, or they will kill you," Angelo told Angelina.

The couple returned to the restaurant, and Angelo shot and killed the two strangers. Romanoff then told the couple that they ought to kill themselves. Angelina swallowed vaginal suppositories, perfume, and allergy pills. She did not die. The police traced the couple to their apartment. They were arrested and admitted to a psychiatric hospital.

The case of Angelo and Angelina was described in the *Jefferson Journal of Psychiatry* (January 1993) by Ryan M. Nishihara and Craig T. Nakamura from John A. Burns School of Medicine in Honolulu, Hawaii. It is one of dozens of cases of *Folie-a-Deux,* French for "madness-of-two," a rare psychiatric syndrome in which delusional beliefs and sometimes hallucinations are transferred from one individual to another.

The case of Angelina and Angelo is an extreme example of how your spouse can influence the way you think and behave. A recent article in *Obesity* brings about another example—a milder, more benign one. Here, your spouse's way of thinking and behavior will not end with a murder. Instead, it may result in mild weight loss. I call it *La Diete-a-Deux*.

Amy A. Gorin and her colleagues, working at the Department of Psychological Sciences at the University of Connecticut, sought to answer the question: If one spouse participates in a weight loss program, does the other spouse lose weight?

The authors of the study call this phenomenon—where non-dieting spouses lose weight while their spouses go on a diet—a "ripple effect." The study was supported by Weight Watchers International, Inc.

130 couples participated in Gorin's study. The researchers randomly assigned one member of each couple into two groups. 65 participants were assigned to a Weight Watchers diet (WW) and received 6 months of free access to WW meetings and online tools. The other 65 participants received a 4-page weight loss handout with basic information regarding healthy eating and physical activity. They did not participate in meetings and did not have access to Weight Watchers' online tools.

The spouses of the 130 participants received no treatment at all: no Weight Watchers meeting, no online tools, not even a 4-page weight loss handout.

Most of the couples were married (93.1%); the other couples just lived together.

At 6 months after they embarked on their diet, the participants who were on a WW diet lost more weight than those on the self-guided diet. WW dieters lost 4.31 kgs, while self-guided dieters lost only 3.08 kgs.

Surprisingly, the spouses of the participants also lost weight. At 6 months, spouses of participants on the WW diet lost 2.16 kgs, while spouses on the self-guided diet lost 1.88 kgs. Overall, 32% of the untreated spouses lost 3% or more of their initial body weight.

The study, the authors say, shows that a "ripple effect" does exist and that "weight loss can spread within couples."

From *Folie-a-Deux* to *La Diete-a-Deux:* your spouse's thinking and behavior may have a ripple-effect on your health. As to tips on how to choose the right spouse, I will update you as soon as these become available. Please don't hold your breath.

LA BELLA LUNA

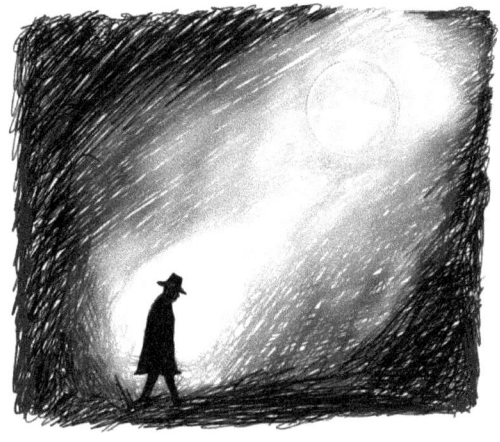

"Loretta, I love you," says Ronny Cammareri (played by Nicolas Cage) in *Moonstruck*, a 1987 movie by Norman Jewison. Ronny continues: "[It is] not like they told you love is ... love don't make things nice - it ruins everything. It breaks your heart. It makes things a mess. We aren't here to make things perfect. The snowflakes are perfect. The stars are perfect. Not us. Not us! We are here to ruin ourselves and to break our hearts and love the wrong people and die. The story books are bullshit."

Moonstruck's original title was *The Bride and the Wolf*, but Jewison, the director, felt that *Moonstruck* was a better name, because the movie is "about the moon. Everybody's talking about the moon. The father's talking about the moon, the full moon. We keep shooting the moon ... So we called it *Moonstruck*."

In *Moonstruck*, under the full moon, love strikes with ferocity.

The influence of the moon is not limited to its effect on love. In Shakespeare's play, for example, when Othello is informed about foul murders that were committed, Othello responds: "It is the very error of the moon; She comes more nearer earth than she was wont, And makes men mad."

Whether it be moonstruck lovers, the sinking of the Titanic, or foul murders, the moon has often been implicated as a co-conspirator. Even the word 'lunatic,' used to describe the mentally ill, the extremely foolish, and the eccentric, is derived from luna, Latin for 'moon.'

So, on a dark night in December (the moon wasn't full, I swear), I asked myself: what else could the moon, full or eclipsed, be blamed for?

In the entertaining Christmas 2017 issue of the prestigious and very serious *British Medical Journal*, I found a surprising article. Donald A. Redelmeier from the Department of Medicine at the University of Toronto and Eldad Shafir from the Department of Psychology at Princeton University examined the question: does a full moon contribute to motorcycle-related death?

Redelmeier and Shafir report that motorcycle crashes in the US account for nearly 5000 deaths a year and that the average motorcyclist faces a greater risk of death than a drunk driver without a seatbelt.

Redelmeier and Shafir analyzed safety data from the US Highway Traffic Safety Administration. They included information from January 1975 to December 2014, with a total of 494 full moon nights (typically one or two nights a month). They compared the rates of motorcycle-related deaths during full moon nights to mortality during the nights one week before and one week after a full moon (the control group).

The authors found that a total of 13,029 people were killed in motorcycle crashes during 1,482 nights (494 full moon nights and 988 control nights).

The typical motorcyclist-victim was a middle-aged man riding a street bike with a large engine in a rural location. Fewer than half of the victims were wearing a helmet.

The authors found that the risk of fatal motorcycle accidents was greater on nights with a full moon (9.1 fatal crashes per night occurred on full moon nights, compared with 8.64 on nights without a full moon). The risk of fatal crashes was even greater during supermoon nights, when the moon was about 50,000 kilometers closer to Earth and its light brighter.

Similar results were seen in the United Kingdom, Canada, and Australia.

How do the authors explain the association between the full moon and the increased risk of fatal motorcycle accidents?

Perhaps it is because the full moon travelers ride their motorcycles more often, faster, or farther. Perhaps it is because on these nights with a full moon, the travelers' hearts follow a road less travelled, or a route less familiar.

But a different explanation is more plausible: "A full moon," the authors write, "is infrequent and spectacular..." The full moon is large and bright against a dark sky. It can appear abruptly between buildings, past trees, and over hills. It engenders wonderment and awe. In short, a full moon is a natural distraction.

I wanted to write to Redelmeier and Shafir and ask them to examine the correlations between a full moon and other aspects of life. Is there truth in Shakespeare's observation that when the moon "comes more nearer earth ... " it makes men mad? Was the old man in *Moonstruck* right when he looked at the moon and declared: "La bella luna! The moon brings the woman to the man."

I wanted to ask Redelmeier and Shafir whether men and women are destined to be distracted, forever searching the sky for answers, always looking at the moon for clues, yearning to mend their hearts, untangle the mess, and love the right people.

THE DIVORCE PARTY

"Jeff Bezos throws celebrity-packed party at his NYC apartment 8 months after finalizing divorce." *AOL.com*

Celebrations of beginnings and endings occur often and everywhere: high-school graduations and commencement parties, baby showers and funerals, bachelor parties and weddings. The other day, after I had read about Jeff Bezos' party, I asked myself, 'Why wasn't I ever invited to a divorce party?'

Devoid of any real-life experience in partying with divorcees, I couldn't even imagine what a divorce party might look like. 'A good starting point,' I thought, 'would be to first reflect on weddings instead.'

So I imagined a wedding: the bride is glowing with happiness in a fancy, white dress. The groom is well-groomed and smiling in a meticulously tailored suit and tie. The bride's mother is crying happy tears. The guests are polite, carrying gifts in envelopes and packages. A three course meal; chicken, steak, or fish; red or white wine. A tall, three-tier wedding cake. A band that rocks the dancing floor. A photographer is taking pictures, for posterity. A priest, or a rabbi, and a ring. And a promise: to have and to hold, from this day forward, for better, for worse, for richer, for poorer, in sickness and in health, until death do us apart.

This exercise of my imagination felt so good that in order to remain realistic, I just had to remind myself of the bitter truth. For some couples, marriage isn't as advertised. Disillusion and disagreements arise, bickering and quarrels develop, and promises are broken. And by the numbers, according to the US Census bureau (2009 data), by the age of 50, more than one third of all adults will be divorced.

After imagining a wedding and reading the grim statistics, it became easier for me to imagine a divorce party. 'It could look almost like a wedding,' I thought: the past bride, in a fancy dress (color of her choice). The former groom, well-groomed, in a meticulously tailored suit and tie (also color of her choice). The bride's mother is crying. The guests are polite and understanding. The wedding gifts, or cash equivalent, are returned to the givers. A three course meal; chicken, steak, or fish; red or white wine. A cake. A band that rocks the dancing floor. A photographer is taking pictures, for posterity. No priest, nor a rabbi. And no ring returned (you earned it, honey).

Why wasn't I ever invited to a divorce party? As I was searching the medical literature for clues, I found a study that was published in the journal *Circulation* showing that divorce is a significant risk factor for the development of a heart attack (acute myocardial infarction, or AMI).

The author, Matthew E. Dupre, and his colleagues from Duke University, followed a group of 15,827 married and divorced individuals, 45 to 80 years old, for 18 years. More than one third of the group members were divorced at least once. Overall, the rates of AMI were higher among those who were divorced. The risk of developing AMI was 1.24 times higher in women who had one divorce, and 1.77 times higher in women who were divorced twice or more. Even in women who remarried, the risk of developing AMI remained 1.35 times higher than in the continuously married women. In other words, remarried women had similar risks for the development of AMI as divorced women.

Men proved more resilient. The risk of AMI increased only in men with a history of two or more divorces (1.3 times the chance of developing AMI), and men who remarried had no significant additional risk.

Why is divorce associated with a higher risk of AMI? The prevailing argument is that divorce has a negative impact on the economic, behavioral, and emotional well-being of individuals and consequently on their ability to prevent, detect, and treat illness. A more detailed analysis of Dupre's data, however, led the authors to a different conclusion: they suspected that the biological effects of acute and chronic stress associated with divorce is the cause of the increased risk of AMI. Interestingly, separate studies found that other social stressors, such as job loss and unemployment, have an effect similar to that of divorce on the risk of AMI.

Why wasn't I ever invited to a divorce party? It is mainly because divorce parties are rare. Matthew E. Dupre, the researcher from Duke University, would suggest, perhaps, that it is hard to genuinely celebrate a life event associated with dire consequences such as a heart attack. I suspect, though, that the reason is different: the promise, to have and to hold . . . until death do us apart, isn't just a promise, it is an ideal, a dream of love, marriage, and living happily-ever-after. Even if it is a dream-come-true to only a few, it is still a dream shared by many. And when a dream comes crushing down, there is no cause for celebration.

COLLECTIVE WISDOM

Imagine that you are a doctor, someone like Dr. House on the popular television show. Your patients believe that you know it all. Your colleagues consider you an expert. You are not particularly humble, but you are honest enough to admit, at least to yourself, that you know *almost* everything, for there would always be a medical case you couldn't solve, or a patient whose medical condition would leave you puzzled.

Suppose you have admitted a patient to your service. Her name is Elizabeth. She is 13 years old and has a disease called Systemic *Lupus* Erythematosus (SLE). You quickly remind yourself of all you have ever learned about the condition: SLE is an autoimmune disease, a condition in which the immune system mistakenly identifies a part of the body as being foreign and attacks its own cells. It can affect almost any part of the body at any time. It behaves in unpredictable ways, with periods of exacerbations and remissions. It can mimic other conditions and confuse the best of doctors. You also know that in some patients with SLE, the immune system attacks the skin, creating a typical reddish rash on the cheeks that resembles a butterfly, or the pattern of fur on a wolf's face, hence the name 'Systemic Lupus Erythematosus' (Lupus is Latin for 'wolf'; *Erythro* is Greek for 'red').

Imagine the healthy Elizabeth. Use a soft brush and

paint her on your mental canvas: her hair red, her smile wide. With a sharp pencil, add several happy freckles to her cheeks.

But on the day Elizabeth was admitted to the hospital, Elizabeth was pale and frightened, her smile erased. Her blood test results were ominous. You noticed that her immune system had chosen a new target, her pancreas. She was seriously ill. And if you would have listened carefully, beyond the usual hum of a busy hospital, you would have heard her asking her mother a question the answer to which you would not know: "Mommy, am I going to die?"

A report on a case similar to the one I just described was published in the New England Journal of Medicine. The patient, a 13-year-old girl who had been previously diagnosed with SLE, was admitted to the hospital in a critical state. Her doctors were concerned that her condition would become complicated by thrombosis (formation of blood clots inside blood vessels). They considered the use of anticoagulation (blood thinners) to prevent the formation of thrombosis, but they were facing a dilemma: if they withheld anticoagulation, she could indeed develop thrombosis, but if they were to treat the patient with anticoagulation, she could end up bleeding profusely. Under usual circumstances, these doctors would consult a textbook, journal articles, or their colleagues. Unfortunately, there was very little knowledge of the use of anticoagulation in critically ill children with SLE.

The doctors needed to decide swiftly, and so they took

an innovative approach. Using a sophisticated search engine, they skimmed through a group of pediatric patients with SLE whose data was stored on the institution's electronic medical record system. Using relevant keywords, the doctors identified ten patients with a condition similar to that of their 13-year-old patient. They reviewed the treatment provided to these patients and analyzed the outcomes. Based on what they learned, they chose to treat the patient with anticoagulation. The patient did well. She did not develop thrombosis, nor did she bleed. She was discharged home in good condition.

In this case, doctors learned from the way other doctors had treated patients with a similar medical problem. By reviewing and adding up the individual experiences of several doctors, they formed a collection of experiences relevant to the case in question, a collective wisdom.

The other day, I entertained myself by asking if a similar approach would work in making decisions regarding romantic relationships.

Imagine that you and your romantic partner are facing a fork in the road where you have to make an important decision regarding your love life. I am talking about a critical decision, such as "Should we stay together, or is it time for us to go our separate ways?"

You could rely on professional advice, or discuss your predicament with a close friend, but you suspect that such advice would lack a deep understanding of your unique situation.

But suppose you could tap into an immense database of variables that could inform your decision. It includes factors such as partner age, physical attributes, levels of education and income, family backgrounds, character traits, and the compatibility of future plans. The database also includes information regarding the outcomes of the decisions that have been made by couples like you, in terms of satisfaction and happiness. You and your partner can enter your own data into the computer with a total guarantee that your information would remain private. A few seconds after entering your information, you receive a recommendation based on the experience of many other couples in your situation (Stay Together! Or, Go Your Separate Ways!). The result would also include a statistical prediction regarding the probability and degree of your happiness were you to follow the recommendation. The algorithm used by the system has already been tested and proved reliable, with a high degree of accuracy in predicting the outcomes of relationships just like yours.

But imagine that the system's recommendation doesn't match your own gut feeling. The recommendation is that you should separate from your partner, but you feel that you should stay together, or vice versa. Would you rely on your own decision-making process, your own gut feeling, or would you follow a recommendation based on the experiences of many other couples, a collective wisdom?

PLEASE, HONEY, DON'T TREAT ME LIKE A COMMA

Please, Honey, don't treat me like a comma.
You can write me a sentence, if you wish,
as in 'I love you,'
with a strong subject and a moving verb,
and a period at the end.
Just like this.

You can write me a paragraph in a story of war.
A knight in armor, on a horse.
I will fight for you, day and night,
until death parts us.

You can write me a book, if you wish,
a hard cover embracing a gentle soul.
Yes! Tell me a story of serendipity,
a voyage from seashore to midland,
and how life shaped me from a rough rock
into a river pebble, too smooth to grasp.

If you must, mark me a question,
point at me in exclamation.
A comma would make it all too obvious,
and I want you to always wonder,
for the moment you solve me,
I am an unwanted puzzle, in a crumbled box,
with a missing piece in my heart.

BIOLOGY

TAKE LOVE TWICE DAILY

Shall I compare thee to a summer's day?[1]
My words have no voice,
my similes are empty,
my metaphors pale,
my lines refuse to sculpture your beauty.
At the end of this poem,
I listen to your heart, then to mine,
a rushing rate, irregular rhythm,
Tick-tock, tick-tock, tick ... tock.

My love for you isn't aimless.[2]
At the end of this poem,
I feel for your pulse, then for mine,
a flow so full, purposeful,
Love-dub, love-dub, love-dub.

In the theater of dreams,
lights on, the curtains withdrawn,
gloves and scrubs,

I pour sleep into your veins,
I weave a common thread through your stories,
and turn into dust the boulders that break your rivers,[3]
I replace your heart valves with smooth velvet,
    so your love flows in my direction,[4]
and mend your broken wing, leaving a crack,
    so your love stays with me.
At the end of this poem,
I write for you, then for me,
Take Love Twice Daily.

References:

1. Burrow, Colin, ed. (2002). *The Complete Sonnets and Poems*. The Oxford Shakespeare. Oxford: Oxford University Press. ISBN 978-0192819338. OCLC 48532938.

2. Billy Collins. Aimless Love: *New and Selected Poems*. Random House. 2013.

3. Aldoukhi AH, Black KM, Ghani KR. *Emerging Laser Techniques for the Management of Stones*. Urol Clin North Am. 2019;46(2):193-205.

4. Star A. *A cherry blossom moment in the history of heart valve replacement*. J Thorac Cardiovasc Surg. 2010;140(6):1226-9.

THE OTHER GIRL WITH THE DRAGON TATTOO

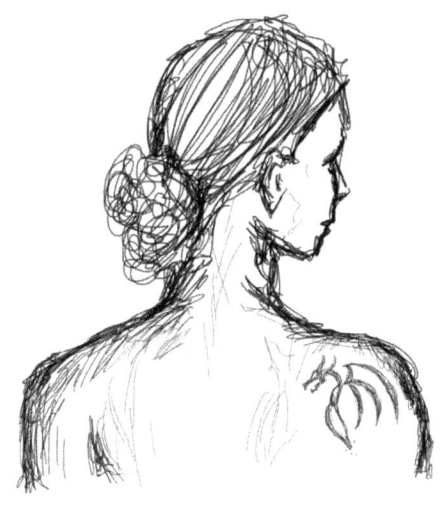

Chuck and Vera spent their second date at Antoni's. They shared the gnocchi in marinara sauce, then a pizza with anchovies, and when the time came for "a tiramisu with two spoons, por favore," he couldn't but realize that he was in love. Vera was his type, more so than any other woman. She was fit, witty, and her smile was smashing. They sat at a narrow table across from each other, their knees touching, holding hands. Vera was wearing a dress that revealed her shoulders. Chuck noticed a tattoo etched on her right shoulder.

"Is that a dragon?" Chuck asked, as he looked at the beast breathing fire out of its nostrils.

"It is," she said.

"Why a dragon?" he asked. "And why is the dragon missing a tail?"

"I tell the story of my life by etching tattoos on my body," Vera said.

"A story of a dragon with a missing tail! Please, I beg you, tell me more."

"Everyone is missing something," Vera told Chuck, "some are missing a piece of their heart, others lose their mind, and a dragon, an angry dragon with a fire in its belly, may miss a tail."

"Are you the girl with the dragon tattoo, like in the book?" he asked.

"I have a story that reads like a book," Vera said, "but I would rather keep it to myself. People might call it a secret, but, to me, I am just practicing being mysterious. I noticed that men like mysterious women. Don't they?" She did not wait for him to answer. "Can you handle a girl who carries around secrets etched on her skin?"

"Of course I can, baby," Chuck said, "of course I can."

Eight months later Vera and Chuck got married. And three years after they got married—Vera was 31 at the time—she arrived at the fertility clinic at a large university hospital.

"When I was 16," Vera told the doctor, "my mother took me to the clinic. I was sixteen and still didn't get my period. My mother was concerned. They told my mother that I do not have a uterus, and that I would never be able to become pregnant." As she told her story, Vera remembered how her mother—a cold woman who saw life as a sequence of inconvenient moments—took her aside and sat with her on a bench in a long, seemingly endless hospital corridor. She remembered her mother's words: "Darling, my darling, you are missing a part, the doctor told me that you don't have a uterus, and if you want someone to love you, anyone, you would better keep it a secret!"

The doctor at the fertility clinic examined Vera. He found Vera to be tall and thin. He noticed that Vera lacked body hair and that her hands were bigger than normal. She appeared feminine and her breasts were normal. On pelvic exam he could not find a uterus.

Two weeks later when the results of her blood tests and imaging studies were back, Vera met with the doctor again. "What your doctor told you at age 16 is right," the doctor told Vera. "When I examined you, I couldn't feel a uterus, nor ovaries. This is the reason you never had a menstrual period. This is one of the reasons you can't get pregnant.

"The imaging study you had—the MRI—confirms that you don't have a uterus. Your blood work shows a level of testosterone that is very high. And", the doctor continued, as his portrayal of the diagnosis became more ominous with each sentence, "your genetic testing shows that you have an X-chromosome and a Y-chromosome. Normally, a woman would have two X-chromosomes. In other words, you have the genetic constitution of a man, not a woman."

Back at home, Chuck was still at work, and Vera had the whole apartment to herself. She took a hot shower in an attempt to wash her thoughts away. Yet, she saw herself as the child she once was, at 16, receiving the bad news about a medical condition she couldn't understand. She saw, in her mind, the days that followed—the declining grades at school, the partying, the men she dated as if to heal a wound that would never heal, the visit to "Ink — Tattoos for Life," where she asked a man with a long beard and a steady hand to etch a dragon in her own image, with an angry fire and a missing tail.

She also remembered good moments from her recent days and weeks, with Chuck, her husband, who showed her true love. 'How did it all happen?' she wondered. 'What will become of me, of Chuck, of us?' And the most dreaded of all questions quickly formed in her mind: 'Am I a woman or a man?'

Here is how doctors think. Whether a person will become a man or a woman is determined by a series of fateful, dramatic events that take place well before birth. Doctors call the process where the sex of a person is determined 'sexual differentiation.' It happens like this: In the fetus, both men and women have primitive gonads—these are the anatomical structures that later turn into either testes (male gonads) or into ovaries (female gonads). Men have an X-chromosome and a Y-chromosome. Women have two X-chromosomes (and no

Y-chromosome). The process of sexual differentiation is signaled by a gene on the Y-chromosome. This gene, the SRY gene ('SRY' for 'sex-determining region of the Y'), carries the information—encoded in its DNA molecules—necessary for the gonads to develop into testes. The testes produce testosterone, which signals the development of the Wolffian duct, from which the typical male genitalia develop. In the absence of a Y-chromosome, a different process ensues: the gonads develop into ovaries, and the typical female phenotype develops with fallopian tubes, a uterus, and a vagina.

Vera was looking for an explanation for her condition, perhaps even a solution. Her doctors translated her quest into a simple question: what has gone awry in Vera's process of sexual differentiation?

Encountered with any complex medical riddle, doctors go into a "differential diagnosis" mode. They ask themselves what the causes for a condition might be, and then, by way of elimination, or deduction, they arrive at the most likely explanation.

Vera's condition could have been the result of a defect in the synthesis of testosterone. The body produces testosterone in a rather complex process. Any defect in the enzymes participating in testosterone production could lead to a lack of testosterone and altered sexual differentiation. But Vera's testosterone levels were high.

Vera's condition could have been the result of a defect in the development of her Müllerian duct (the structure that develop into the fallopian tubes, uterus, cervix and the upper part of the vagina). But patients with that condition—called the Mayer–Rokitansky–Küster–Hauser syndrome—do have ovaries, and when they hit puberty their breasts develop, and hair grows in their pubic area and in their armpits. Vera did not have normal ovaries (a surgery her doctors performed to remove her gonads revealed testes instead). And she lacked pubic hair.

The doctors considered other diagnoses, but only one diagnosis could explain Vera's condition. It is called Androgen (or Testosterone) Insensitivity Syndrome. Normally, testosterone would be produced in the gonads and released into the blood stream. It would then attach to a specific receptor (an androgen receptor) in the cells in its target tissues and "tell" the cells what they should "do" and how they should "behave."

Patients, like Vera, with Androgen Insensitivity Syndrome have an X-chromosome and a Y-chromosome like a normal man would have. Their gonads are producing testosterone like in a normal man. But due to a mutation in the gene that encodes for the receptor for testosterone, the message that would normally be delivered by testosterone does not translate into a proper response. The Wolffian duct doesn't develop, and patients end up having female-appearing external genitalia but no uterus.

The news hit Vera hard. Her initial response was to never tell her husband. But then, once several days had passed, the truth became a burden she could no longer carry alone. She called Chuck, her husband, to the living room. "I have something to tell you," she said, and then continued her story. Chuck listened. He saw the pain in Vera's eyes. He told her he accepted her the way she is, and that no matter what her chromosomes say, she is as much of a woman as she had always been.

Through an in-vitro fertilization (using an egg from an egg-donor) and a surrogate carrier (a woman who carried and delivered the baby), Vera and Chuck had a baby girl.

A year later, Vera returned to "Ink — Tattoos for Life." The man who etched the dragon tattoo on her right shoulder was no longer working there. "Can you add a tail to my dragon?" She asked the woman at the front desk. She felt whole as a woman, and she wanted her dragon tattoo to reflect just that.

POTS AND LIDS

My grandmother was the queen of sayings. One day, after she served vanilla, chocolate, and strawberry ice cream, for *"variety is the spice of life,"* she misinterpreted my postprandial sluggishness as a sign of concern over my prospects of finding the right woman. "Don't worry," she said in her usual, comforting tone, "every pot has its lid."

But if women and men are the pots and lids of dating, the world is a kitchen from hell. I saw pots and lids everywhere! Big pots, small pots, tall and short, heavy and light. Some pots were cast-iron and built to last, while others had non-stick personalities. Some pots were perfectly composed, yet others were crooked, dented at the rim, or missing a love handle. My kitchen was a chaotic disarray of lonely pots and lids, unlikely to find a proper fit, let alone cook happily ever after.

Attempts to properly pair lonely hearts are almost as old as history itself. At first, arranged marriage seemed to be an elegant solution. After all, who in their right mind would put the delicate task of romantic matching in the hands of inexperienced youngsters? It worked quite well, almost everywhere in the world, until the 18th century when ideas such as individualism and social mobility started to develop. Young people suddenly had strong feelings and original opinions, and the seemingly logical solution of arranged marriage began to crumble.

Romantic matching then evolved in the name of freedom, equality, the pursuit of happiness, and preference for randomness. People fell for each other everywhere and at all times. They met in high school, in college, around the water cooler at work, and serendipitously on the streets and in bars. They matched spontaneously and abruptly, without prior examination, proper planning, or expert advice.

The latest attempt at matching takes no such random chances and has no geographical limits. Spread over more than 150 countries, the members of eHarmony.com, for example, are matched based on their responses to a long questionnaire and a long list of other variables. A complex matching algorithm is then used to optimize the chance for long-term relationships.

No matter what matching system is used, the results are not uniformly satisfactory and too often, tears are shed, hearts are broken, and the "and-they-lived-happily-ever-after" fairy tales painfully collapse.

Why then do we continue? Because reproduction is nature's command, a pre-requisite for survival as a species. Women and men do not just wish to match. Like all other living organisms—from bacteria to mammals—humans are programmed to reproduce.

And we come prepared for the task of reproduction. Women and men are equipped with complementary reproductive systems and an intense drive, fueled by a relentless endocrine system, to procreate. These forces work together toward a biologically desirable rendezvous between a sperm cell (spermatozoon) and an egg (ovum), a moment of fertilization, the creation of a new life.

The story of fertilization is even more precarious than the story of matching. It is an epic of survival in the face of unfavorable odds. During sexual intercourse, about 300 million sperm cells enter the vagina, but only one spermatozoon will reach its final destination and fertilize the egg. The rest will perish in one of many ways: some will succumb upon impact with the acidic environment of the vagina; others will be identified as foreign invaders, engulfed and enzymatically destroyed by cells of the female immune system; half of the remaining spermatozoa will find themselves in a dead-end, for only one of the two fallopian tubes contain the desirable egg. A few dozen cells will eventually reach the egg. The first spermatozoon to enter the egg, the sole survivor, will fertilize the egg in a swift, winner-takes-all victory.

This whole process of sexual reproduction is cumbersome, heart breaking, wasteful. Every pot may have its lid, but boy is it difficult to find a match. Why does the story of fertilization need to be so complex, so heroic? Couldn't we just reproduce asexually as bacteria do, by splitting into two? Wouldn't it be simpler if we could just do as bakers' yeast cells do and peacefully bud off from one another?

From a biological standpoint, sexual reproduction, although more complex, offers a significant advantage over asexual reproduction, for it combines the genetic material of two different organisms. Whereas asexual reproduction results in large colonies of identical individuals, in sexual reproduction the offspring are genetically different from their parents, exhibiting diverse traits and characteristics, allowing them to better adapt to a changing environment, increasing their chances of survival.

Sexual reproduction is also more fun (and not just because of the process itself), for the result is a society filled with different pots and lids, crowded with interesting characters. After all, my grandmother was right: variety is the spice of life!

MEN ARE FROM EARTH, WOMEN ARE FROM EARTH

How different are women from men? So different, claims John Gray, an author and relationship guru, that the two sexes seem to have come from different planets. His book "Men are from Mars, Women are from Venus," published in 1993 by HarperCollins, became a bestseller (more than 50 million copies sold) and has influenced how women and men view themselves and the opposite sex.

In the world according to Gray, when women bring up a problem in a conversation, for example, they merely want to talk about it, not necessarily solve it. Men, on the other hand, are so eager to come up with solutions to the problem that they totally fail to listen. Then, the woman says, "You don't ever listen," and he responds with "You don't understand," and she concludes that "You don't love me anymore." He retreats to his man-cave (nowadays, the garage), while she still yearns for connection. And things go south.

Some critics say that "Men are from Mars, Women are from Venus" is overly simplistic, excessively stereotypical, and based on opinions rather than on scientific research.

Does scientific research support the claims made in "Men are From Mars, Women are from Venus"? Professor Daphna Joel from Tel Aviv University and her colleagues looked at how different male brains are from female brains.

The authors looked at MRIs (Magnetic Resonance Imaging studies) of more than 1,400 human brains. Unlike researchers before them, Joel and her colleagues did not look at the difference between men and women in a single brain element. Instead, they identified 10 regions in the brain showing the largest sex differences. They looked at the grey matter, white matter, and at measures of connectivity between different brain areas. Looking at these regions, they found extensive overlap between the structures of the brain in men and women. They found that most brains were comprised of mosaics of features, some more common in men and some more common in women.

The authors also analyzed two large databases that included information on many psychological variables for a large number of subjects. These variables included measures of behavior, personality characteristics, and attitudes. Using statistical analyses similar to the ones used to analyze the data obtained from the MRIs, they identified seven variables with the largest sex differences. Again, substantial variability was evident in 59% of the study participants. Only a few study participants exhibited internal consistency (having exclusively female or male features).

Joel and her colleagues concluded that although there are some sex differences in brain structure between men and women, brains do not fall into a binary of female or male, and they are not even aligned along a male—female brain continuum. "Each brain is a unique mosaic of features," they claimed, "some of which may be more common in females compared with males, others may be more common in males compared with females, and still others may be common in both females and males."

Similarly, their analyses of gender-related data revealed extensive overlap between females and males in personality traits, attitudes, interests, and behaviors.

I wonder: does Joel's study prove that men aren't from Mars, women aren't from Venus, and that they should just live happily ever after here, on Earth? Perhaps the differences between the sexes are beyond the resolution of an MRI scan, a difference in how individual groups of brain cells work, in the way these cells communicate with each other, in the way they respond to the different hormonal environments in men and women. Similarly, could it be that the gender-related data that Joel's study analyzed was not specific enough to identify the profound differences that make people believe that men are from Mars, that women are from Venus?

In the Customer Review section on Amazon.com I read, with great interest, a review of "Men are from Mars, Women are from Venus." It was written by a man who holds a degree in rocket engineering. His review indicates that he has been in dire need of a self-help book that would help him decipher the mysteries of the opposite sex. He writes: "The book is the equivalent of

'The Idiot's guide to Listening, Respect, and Communication,' with Easy-to-Remember Examples." And still, he recommends the book, because "I don't want to know the fundamentals of communications, I just want to know why my last girlfriend got offended when I offered solutions when she was complaining about work."

And if he would come to me for advice, I would simply say, "She never wanted your advice. Just listen, man, you have to listen!"

OF MICE AND MEN

When caught in the act of infidelity, cheaters often borrow from the excuses of artful diplomats.

Stephen Walt, a professor of international relations at Harvard University, proposes 21 handy talking-points to defend the indefensible in foreign policy (invading other countries with no provocation, for example). Here are a few:

1. We didn't do it!

2. We know you think we did it, but we aren't admitting to it.

3. Actually, maybe we did do something, but not what we are accused of doing.

4. OK, we did it, but it wasn't that bad.

5. What we did was really quite restrained, when you consider how powerful [or attractive] we are. I mean, we could have done something even worse.

6. Plus, they [you] started it [or, you just don't pay attention to me anymore].

Change 'we' to 'I,' and add 'Honey' at the beginning of each sentence, and these talking-points could serve to help cheaters defend the indefensible.

But wait! There is more. A recent article in the prestigious journal Nature provides one additional talking-point to the list. It has to do with biology and genetics, mice and men. Let me explain.

Andres Bendesky from Harvard University and his colleagues examined the genetic basis of monogamy and parental behavior in mammals. The researchers studied two different species of mice: the promiscuous deer mouse and the monogamous old-field mouse.

Monogamy is an exception in the world of mammals. Only about 5% of mammalian species are monogamous. The old-field male mouse belongs to this group; it forms a long-term bond with one female and offers parental care to his offspring.

Old-field mice and deer mice do not mingle in nature. Each keeps to itself. But when Bendesky placed them in cages, a single deer mouse and a single old-field mouse left alone in a cage, they interbred. Their hybrid offspring were healthy and fertile. The hybrid offspring were then allowed to copulate and have offspring of their own. Five mice from each species (10 parents, first generation) produced 30 hybrid mice (second generation), which then produced 769 offspring of their own (third generation).

Bendesky then compared the parenting behaviors of the different mice groups and of the different generations. He observed parenting behaviors, such as how much parents were licking their pups, how long they huddle their young, the quality of the nests they were building for their pups, and the degree to which they were trying to retrieve their offspring once those were taken away from them.

The monogamous old-field mice demonstrated stronger parenting behaviors than did the promiscuous deer mice. But in the second, and even more so in the third generation, parental behaviors varied widely. Some offspring were as dedicated to their pups as the monogamous old-field mice; some demonstrated only a subset of parental behaviors only part of the time; others had a cavalier attitude toward their offspring – they just didn't give a damn.

The researchers then scanned the DNA of the hybrid mice and found twelve different locations within it, stretches of DNA that were clearly linked to specific parenting behaviors. Eight of these stretches of DNA were sex-specific, affecting male parents and female parents differently.

Bendesky's study was met with enthusiasm. A headline in *The New York Times* read: "Why are Some Mice (and People) Monogamous? A Study Points to Genes."

The study is important, because it demonstrates that, in mice, some parental behaviors are determined by genes.

Cheaters may find Bendesky's study interesting for another reason. It provides another convenient talking-point that they can use to defend their indefensible behavior: "But Honey," the unfaithful would say, "it's not me, it's my genes."

The more cool-minded spouse would then point out that the study was examining parental behaviors, not monogamy or promiscuity. The astute partner would also ask: "And what—are you a mouse?"

WHY IS THE Y DISAPPEARING?

The human Y chromosome is threatening to disappear. It is not the number of copies of the Y chromosome that is in any immediate danger. After all, there is still one copy of the Y chromosome in almost each cell in the male body, or about 30 trillion copies of it in each man. But, the size of the Y chromosome—and I don't know how else to break the news to you—is shrinking.

To put things in order, I would like to remind you that there are 23 pairs of chromosomes in our body. They contain our DNA—the instruction-manual for everything that is going on in our bodies, from the color of our eyes to how fast our hearts beat. One of the 23 pairs is the pair of sex chromosomes. Women have two X chromosomes. Men have one X chromosome and one Y chromosome (I will simply call it 'Y,' pronounced 'why,' as in 'why not?').

Scientists believe that the shrinking of Y began 300,000 years ago when two regular-looking chromosomes decided to specialize. Since then, the X chromosome has preserved 98% of its genetic content. The manly Y, on the other hand, has grown a beard and gone rogue, retaining only 3% of its ancestral genes. And so, if you look closely at the X and Y chromosomes, you will be struck by the difference. The X chromosome looks like all other non-sex chromosomes: two plump hotdogs twisted around each other at the middle, taking the shape of the letter 'X.' On the other hand, Y doesn't look like the letter 'Y' (its name derives from the order in which it was discovered, as in X, Y, Z, not from its shape). Instead, it looks diminished and humbled by a tragic history of loss, a piece of paper crumpled into a little ball. It seems to be of no use or distinction, an undesirable object.

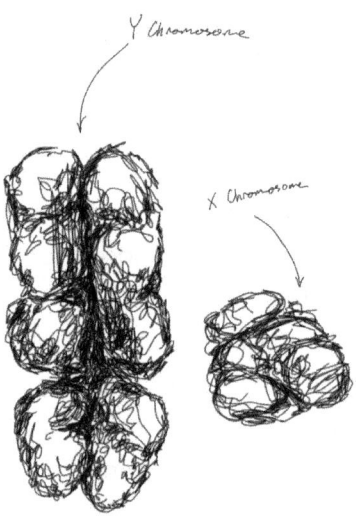

Some women would take comfort in the demise of Y. They might see Y as the source of all trouble, a collection of genes that add no value to the world, that propagate undesired manly traits such as selective hearing ("they never listen"), selective memory ("he didn't remember my birthday"), addiction to TV channel flipping, over-confidence, and hairy ears. Other women, however, might miss the Y and admit that "the sex [chromosome] was great while it lasted."

Scientists try to remain calm. They found that from a genetic standpoint, humans are very similar to each other. Pick any two random men, and you will find that their DNA is 99.9% identical. The same applies to two randomly selected women. If you compare women to men, however, the picture changes dramatically. The DNA of women and men is only 98.5% identical. This 1.5% difference may still seem small, until you consider that the DNA of a human and a chimpanzee is also 98.5% identical. In other words, from a genetic standpoint, my wife's DNA is as close to my DNA as it is to the DNA of a chimpanzee. And please, I beg of you, don't jump to conclusions.

What does this difference between the genetic composition of men and women mean? It is obvious that the genes on Y encode for male-specific characteristics. They determine the sex of the fetus, the formation of testes, and the formation of sperm cells. What is less obvious is this: first, the Y genes are present in almost all somatic cells; and second, these genes affect the development of organs outside of the genital system.

In an article in the *Journal of Proteome Research*, for example, Anna Meyfour and her colleagues described 48 Y-chromosome genes. Most of these genes are related to male-specific characteristics, but some genes have a role in the development of tooth enamel, the kidneys, the heart, even the brain.

For those of us who thought that the differences between men and women stem from different hormonal environments, these findings are a dramatic twist in the plot.

Doctors and scientists have known for a long time that a sea of difference exists between men and women in their tendencies to suffer from different diseases. Four times more men than women are diagnosed with autism-spectrum-disorder. On the other hand, women are more likely to suffer from auto-immune diseases. These differences may be due to different hormonal environments, differences in behaviors (men engage in risky behaviors more often), but some of the differences may be due to the expression of Y-chromosome genes.

According to some scientists, the shrinking Y is expected to completely disappear in exactly 4.6 million years. It leaves ample time to answer questions like: Can better understanding of the Y chromosome and its genes help cure diseases that present differently in men and women? How will a world without Y look like? How are men *really* different from women? And why is Y disappearing?

THE RABBIT

There are two stories that I would like to tell you. The first story is about Ralph A., a 65-year-old school principal in New England who suddenly lost his stream of consciousness. The other story is that of Claude Bernard, a 19th century French physiologist who is considered to be one of the greatest scientists in history. Despite the time difference and the vast geographical distance between the two men, their stories intersect in my mind, for Claude Bernard's observations provide a framework for understanding and solving Ralph's medical mystery.

It was early summer in New England, and Ralph was busy running the local high-school. There was an urgent need to investigate who threw a stone at the teachers' lounge window; Bob's mother wasn't happy about Mrs. Johnson's grading policy ("Bob deserves an A+," she protested); Mr. Peterson, a Math teacher, called in sick at the last moment; and there was no money in the budget for the graduation ceremony. "I am so ready to retire," Ralph thought to himself. He felt exhausted. His head started to ache.

Over the next three weeks, Barbara, Ralph's wife, noticed that something was the matter with him. With each passing day, his fatigue intensified. "True, his morning headaches are mild, and they do slowly disappear after he takes a couple of pills, but who has a headache every single day?" she asked herself. Then Ralph became forgetful ("Is it really your birthday today, Honey?" he asked her). A week later, Ralph became progressively confused—one early morning, she found him stretched, face down, on the loveseat in their living room. He was fully dressed in his suit and shoes, hugging his school briefcase under his chest, his snoring interrupted only by incoherent mumbling that sounded something like "Banana! ... Umbrella! ... Ba-na-na!" It was a Sunday morning, she knew, and Ralph never went to work on Sundays—Barbara realized that it was time for them to go to the Emergency Room.

"There is something wrong with my husband," she told the doctor, "it seems that he lost his stream of consciousness." The doctor asked Ralph a few questions, like "Do you know where you are?" and "Do you know what is today's date?" and "Do you know who I am, and what I am doing here?" Ralph answered correctly. He was oriented to time and place, and he understood that he was in a hospital for a good reason.

"Consciousness forever changes," the doctor told Barbara. "It can ebb and flow."

"It may be," Barbara said, "but lately, doctor, my husband's consciousness only ebbs—it doesn't flow!"

The doctor found out that Ralph's blood pressure was very high (203/102 mm Hg), that his heart was pounding hard and fast, and that he was breathing fast. Nothing else in the physical examination was wrong. 'Perhaps something was amiss?' the doctor thought. But when Ralph's blood tests came back, it became evident that his kidneys were failing. And an imaging study, an MRI of his brain, showed patches of cerebral edema, or, to put it simply, swelling of Ralph's brain. The swelling affected Ralph's white matter and gray matter.

The doctor believed Ralph's wife from the beginning, but now that he saw the images of Ralph's brain on the monitor, he didn't have even a shred of doubt that her story was true—for if the brain is the throne for a man's consciousness, then a swollen, suffering brain would be a reason for a mind lost.

"The findings in the CT scan," the doctor told Barbara, "indicate that your husband has PRES, or posterior reversible encephalopathy syndrome. It means that his brain doesn't look or function the way it should. It could be related to your husband's high blood pressure, but also to other conditions; we just don't know yet. We will run a few more tests, and we will start treating him with medications for hypertension. We believe it might solve the problem," he said.

The blood pressure remained high, and Ralph's consciousness ebbed; it didn't flow.

Barbara was sitting beside her husband's bed. Her mind was swirling with questions: why did Ralph's kidneys fail? Why did his brain suddenly swell? Will he ever again be the Ralph she knew? Will he ever regain his stream of consciousness?

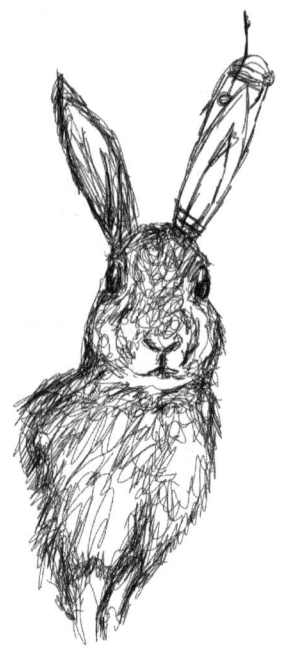

The rabbit lived an uneventful life of no particular consequences until it met the hands of Claude Bernard. Bernard chose the rabbit for its long ears. Bernard was a rotund man with determined eyes and a passion for the study of physiology. On that morning, wearing his white apron, he wrapped each of the rabbit's ears separately and attached to each a device for measuring temperature. He gathered around him a few of his students and several colleagues and called for his assistant. The vivisection—surgery on a living animal—was performed in Bernard's dark, damp laboratory. Bernard held a scalpel and cut through the rabbit's skin. The rabbit whimpered and tried to escape, but it was held still by the assistant. Bernard then cut through the rabbit's muscles and connective tissues, reaching for the rabbit's cervical sympathetic nerve on its left side. He cut the nerve and stimulated it with a needle, on and off, while measuring the temperature in the rabbit's ears. In that particular rabbit experiment, Bernard proved, without any doubt, that stimulating the sympathetic nerve leads to a change in the blood flow to the rabbit's ear—and therefore its temperature.

You might ask: who cares about the temperature in a rabbit's ears? And what happened to Bernard's poor rabbit?

As a young man, the energetic, enthusiastic Claude Bernard (1813-1878) was working as an apprentice in a local pharmacy. He was interested in a career in the theater, but when he showed a play he wrote, *Arthur de Bretagne*, to a renowned critic of the day, the critic shrugged his shoulders and suggested that he try medicine instead. And so, Claude studied medicine with little enthusiasm but found his calling working in the laboratory of François Magendie, a Professor of Medicine at the College de France whose main interest was in physiology. Bernard married Fanny Martin, the daughter of a rich doctor, whom, it seemed, he never loved. Her dowry allowed Bernard to stay in research. Their marriage was long but miserable. If love is an obsession, his was for scientific discovery. Among the many points of contention was Bernard's tendency to bring his work home: He would bring with him some of the animals he studied, cut open and half-alive, with tubes and other devices still stuck in their bodies; he operated on the family dog; he might have even brought the rabbit home, with its ears wrapped, one ear warmer than the other.

In a separate series of experiments, Bernard discovered glycogen—the substance used to store glucose (sugar) in the liver—and showed that stimulation of the vagus nerve would lead to an increase in the level of sugar in the blood and in the urine.

These and other experiments must have led Bernard to have deep thoughts about the complexity with which the body operates. In the rabbit experiment, he could see that a mechanism exists by which the body regulates the blood flow and the temperature of a rabbit's ears. In the liver experiment, he could see that a mechanism exists by which an organism controls its own level of glucose. Bernard must have concluded that there are more mechanisms to control the environment in which our body functions. Bernard must have surmised that these mechanisms keep our internal environment steady. 'But against what?' he must have asked himself. 'Against the ever changing external environment,' was his answer.

About the *milieu intérieur* (French for internal environment), Bernard wrote: "The stability of the internal environment is the condition for the free and independent life."

Bernard was recognized for his accomplishment during his lifetime. Napoléon Bonaparte, the Emperor of France, built for him a laboratory at the Muséum national d'Histoire naturelle. He became a member of the Académie française, and when he died on a cold day in February 1878, he was accorded a public funeral, an honor never before bestowed on a man of science.

Professor Fine was the attending physician caring for Ralph, the 65-year-old school principal who presented to the Emergency Room with progressive fatigue, morning headaches, forgetfulness, and confusion. Professor Fine pushed his heavy glasses up his nose and passed his fingers through his thinning hair. He looked at his computer monitor for clues regarding Ralph's condition. 'What is the matter with Ralph?' he asked himself.

Whenever Professor Fine confronted a challenging medical case (he referred to these cases as riddles), he looked back, for inspiration, to the time when he learned, as a medical student, about Claude Bernard.

It was Claude Bernard, as Professor Fine learned in the History of Medicine class, who noticed through countless experiments and observations that the body maintains a stable internal environment. It was Claude Bernard who understood that keeping the internal environment constant is critical.

During lectures he gave to medical students, Professor Fine explained the different ways the body keeps its own environment stable: "the body uses the nervous system and the hormonal system to regulate itself," he told the students. "It uses sensors to detect changes in the internal environment of the body. The body senses its own temperature and the pressure within its blood vessels, it measures its own state of hydration, it monitors the levels of sodium and glucose, and it keeps track of the acidity of the blood. And then, through a command system, it modulates organs and systems in the body to keep the internal environment stable. In response to increasing levels of glucose, for example, the pancreas would release insulin to bring the level of glucose back to normal. At the same time, the kidneys would clear the blood from toxins and from waste products and take part in maintaining the body's blood pressure, all in the name of keeping every cell exposed to a stable, constant internal environment."

Professor Fine liked to think in those terms because, for him, every disease was a disturbance in the normal balance of the body, a deviation from a steady state. If he could find the cause for that disturbance, if he could correct it and bring the body back to its own stable state of affairs, then the patient would heal, and, just like that, the riddle would be solved!

Confronted with Ralph's deteriorating health, Professor Fine asked himself: 'What is the cause for Ralph's failure to maintain a stable internal environment?'

Ralph's blood pressure was very high (203/102 mm Hg), his heart was pounding hard and fast, and he was breathing fast. Ralph's blood tests indicated that his kidneys were failing. An imaging study, an MRI, of his brain showed patches of cerebral edema, or swelling of the brain. Professor Fine thought that this could be an explanation for Ralph's dire cognitive state.

When Ralph's ultrasound images came back, Professor Fine was finally able to solve the riddle. Ralph's bladder was enormously distended. The bladder usually holds about 300 milliliters of urine, but Ralph's bladder was filled with 2900 milliliters (about a gallon). In Professor Fine's mind, it all became clear. Ralph's prostate was so enlarged that it blocked the channel that drains the bladder. Ralph wasn't able to void efficiently. The pressure within his bladder rose and it back-flowed into his ureters and then to his kidneys. The kidneys could no longer function: they couldn't filter the blood of toxins and waste products, and they couldn't regulate the body's blood pressure. These changes, in turn, must have affected Ralph's brain.

Dr. Goldwater, a urologist, was called to the scene. He stood next to Dr. Fine, and while they examined the ultrasound images, Dr. Goldwater mumbled: "Praise God, King of the Universe, who fashioned Man with wisdom and created within him openings and orifices, pores and hollow passages. And if but one of them were to be ruptured, or but one of them were to be blocked, it would be impossible to survive, and to stand before You."

"Beautifully said," Dr. Fine responded. He knew the ancient Jewish prayer that Dr. Goldwater had just quoted, and he was amazed at how wonderfully it matched his own understanding of the human body. After all, if one opening is closed (in Ralph's case, it would be an enlarged prostate that blocked the urinary flow), how can one maintain a stable environment?

Dr. Goldwater placed a catheter in Ralph's bladder and drained his urine. Later, he took Ralph to the operating room and performed surgery to open the prostatic urethra. After surgery, Ralph was able to void and to empty his bladder. His kidney function returned to normal. Ralph's *milieu intérieur* was balanced and stable again. And his stream of consciousness returned to normal.

SAVING ROMEO: DIARIES OF A TIME TRAVELER

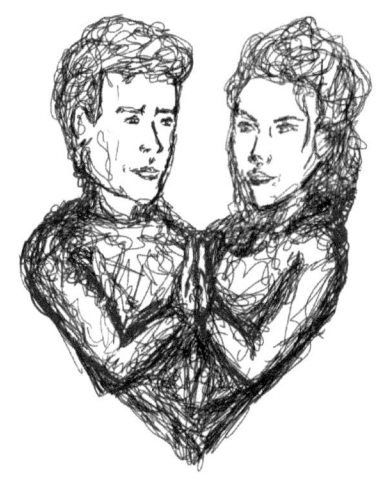

June 16, 2029

As I was reading, for the third time, William Shakespeare's *Romeo and Juliet*, I realized that some love scenes will never die: The scene where Romeo falls for the charming Juliet in the dancing ballroom, for example, or the moment when he stands beneath her balcony enchanted by her beauty, and, perhaps most of all, at the end of the play, the gripping instant when he kneels, heartbroken, beside her body in the crypt. It isn't Shakespeare's dramatic talent only, but also his powerful, poetic language that moves me. I can imagine myself being there, next to Romeo, witnessing the drama: "Did my heart love till now?" he asks, and his answer immediately follows: "Forswear it, Sight! For I ne'er saw true beauty till this night."

And this time, when I read *Romeo and Juliet*, I became convinced that the story must have been real, that *Romeo and Juliet* must have really existed in Verona, Italy. I felt that their love story, the tale of two star-crossed lovers trapped in an impossible relationship must have really taken place, that a tragedy so dramatic, so heartbreaking, could only have come to life as it did in *Romeo and Juliet* if it were true. I thought about Romeo looking at Juliet, mistakenly thinking she was dead, holding the bottle of poison close to his lips. And I thought, 'How unnecessary was Romeo's death? Was it indeed inevitable?'

It isn't just the romantic soul in me that subsequently drove me into action. As a doctor, I can't help but feel that with the latest technology—after all, time traveling has just become commonplace—it is never too late to save a life. I decided to embark on a journey into the past. I wanted to interfere with the events that led to Romeo's death, and I called the mission "Saving Romeo."

July 23, 2029,

I have worked tirelessly to assemble my crew and to prepare our Time Machine Shuttle (TMS-2) for the journey. This morning, I joined Dr. Smith and Dr. Matteo on what would be the journey of a lifetime. Dr. Smith is a geneticist. Dr. Matteo is an expert in linguistics specializing in ancient Italian. Both are good friends. I will be the driver of the TMS-2. Our mission, I reminded everyone, is to save Romeo's life.

A few moments into our time travel mission, we found professor Cardozo hiding behind the rear seat of TMS-2. It was a surprise, because he was never invited. Yes, he was a close friend of ours, but we knew that his vast knowledge of personalized medicine would only interfere with our mission. It was too late for us to go back and leave Cardozo at home, where we thought he belonged, so we insisted that he remain silent, at all times, for any word that might come out of his mouth could jeopardize the mission.

TMS-2 arrived in Verona, Italy, as planned, on a midsummer day in 1591. We arrived at a critical moment. It was several weeks after *Romeo and Juliet* found themselves entangled in an impossible, painful love, and moments before the unfortunate chain of events leading to their death.

Matteo, aided by an ancient map of Verona, quickly led us alongside the Adige river and through the narrow streets of the city. We found Romeo in the tomb. He was holding Juliet in his arms, his tears flooding her hair. We knew that he was under the mistaken impression that Juliet had died. He was holding a bottle from which he was about to drink the poison that would free him from a life not worth living—a life without Juliet.

Looking at Juliet in Romeo's arms, with her eyes closed and her skin pale, I thought: 'I ne'er saw true beauty till that night.' We had no time to admire Juliet's beauty, however. We had to move fast, for TMS-2 was equipped to allow only short visits into the past.

"We are from the future," Matteo told Romeo, "and we are here to save your life." Romeo could probably tell that we were from the future, or at least from a very remote village. Our attire was modern; Matteo had good command of ancient Italian, but his dialect was still different from Romeo's; and we all had blinking and beeping electronic attachments providing us information about our location, the location of TMS-2, the destination time point, and the home time point (which was July 23, 2029, 15:43:38).

Romeo looked at us, his eyes shining with sadness and despair. "How would you even know that my life is in danger?" he asked.

"Your love story became famous," Matteo said. "William Shakespeare himself heard about you, about Juliet, about your impossible love, and he wrote your story, as a wonderful play, so beautiful that everyone knows it. That's how we know that the poison Juliet drank wasn't a poison, that she isn't actually dead, and that you shouldn't kill yourself. In a few moments, she will wake up, and you will be together. All you have to do is wait!"

"Not dead?" Romeo cried out, "look at her, look at my Juliet, her skin is as pale as Death itself, and she doesn't breathe. What else would you call this if not 'Death'?"

Standing there, we were able to understand only a little of the conversation between Matteo and Romeo. We learned about the content of the conversion only later when Matteo filled us in. At the time, we were only able to make out words such as 'William Shakespeare,' 'Dr. Smith,' *'genetica,'* 'Professor Cardozo,' *'futuro,'* 'spaceship,' 'TMS-due,' *'amore,'* and 'Juliet.' Romeo was listening quietly. His expression turned from deep sadness to complete disbelief. Ultimately, Romeo could not be convinced that Juliet was still alive.

In a final, desperate attempt to save Romeo, Dr. Smith, a man of few words, chimed in, and using the admittedly imperfect auto-translator, he said: "Romeo, although I have never been in your situation, I can tell that you are deeply in love, and I can understand your pain. You feel that Juliet's true beauty compares to none, and that you will never be able to find love other than your love for her. But your feelings are based on a misunderstanding of life and a misconception of love. You see," Dr. Smith continued, "in the future, we have found that our body is built of small units called cells. You can't see cells—they are too small—but they are the building blocks of our body, the way cobblestones are used to pave roads. We also learned that within each cell lies a code—we call it "DNA"—which is like a secret language. There are only four letters in this language, but these letters form long words and ultimately a long book that is six billion letters long, a million times the number of stars you can see in the skies! These letters tell a story. They determine whether our eyes are brown or blue and whether our hair is black or golden; they dictate how our body works; they affect how we think and how we feel and how we behave. This genetic code also determines with whom you fall in love."

I suspected that Romeo might have lost his train of thought (I almost did), but the word 'love' seemed to get his attention. Encouraged by Romeo's reaction, Dr. Smith said: "Each of us, including Juliet, has a different code. This is what makes us unique (Romeo nodded agreeably). But Juliet's DNA is only slightly different from that of any other girl you might meet. In fact, only one in a 1,000 letters in her DNA will be different! You see, Romeo," Dr. Smith concluded, "'love is a gross exaggeration of the difference between one person and everybody else' [he used George Bernard Shaw's words naturally, as if they were his own]. And now that you know how similar we humans are, how similar all women are, you must realize that death is too irreversible a choice for you. Death is just too fatal. You must, you must, put this bottle of poison down. You must choose life!" Romeo lowered his arm, but he was still holding the poison. He didn't look completely convinced. "You could love again," Dr. Smith continued, "even if you believe that Juliet is no longer alive, you could love again. If it won't be Juliet, it will be someone else, not too different, at least not from a genetic standpoint."

Dr. Smith's lecture made Professor Cardozo, an expert in personalized medicine, upset. The vein running down his forehead became engorged, and his face turned red. We were afraid that if he were to say anything, he would do so in a professorial tone and in a wholly convincing manner. He would tell Romeo something like: "saying that all girls are almost the same just because they all share an almost identical genetic code is like saying that all books are identical just because they are written using the same letters. And yet, each book tells a different story, and each of us is a unique experiment of nature."

Cardozo would also say (the man is hard to control, he can't stop talking) that the field of personalized medicine actually makes use of these seemingly small, yet important genetic differences. And he would add that personalized medicine has proven that it can deliver the right care, to the right patient, at the right time. No more "one size fits all"! We have already mapped the entire human genome (the Human Genome Project, 2003), he would point out. We can now look at each individual's molecular constitution, their specific DNA, their unique proteins, and predict which diseases they will have and what treatment would fit them best. Cardozo would give examples of achievements in personalized medicine, in the treatment of breast cancer, colon cancer, and many other diseases. Each of us is different, unique, one of a kind, Cardozo would insist.

Luckily, though, Cardozo said nothing. First, he had promised to remain silent at all times, and he had always been a man of his word. Then, there was the time factor: the signals from TMS-2, beeping sounds and blinking lights, intensified, warning us that we had to return to the time machine shuttle fast, or else we would be stuck in Verona, Italy, 1591.

July 24, 2029

We are back at home. We are safe. But what was the fate of Romeo? Did he drink the poison? Did we save his life? I ran to my home library downstairs and opened *The Complete Works of William Shakespeare*. In between *King Lear* and *Macbeth*, I found the story of *Romeo and Juliet* as complete as I had left it. Not even a word had been changed! I realized that our mission to save Romeo had failed. Romeo died; his story kept on living. This realization stirred mixed emotions in my heart. On the one hand, I was happy that future generations would still be able to cry over the scenes of *Romeo and Juliet*. But I was also disappointed in time-traveling's inability to change the past, and in our failed mission to save Romeo's life. I found comfort in the words of my neighbors, the people of the Upper Peninsula of Michigan, who often say "it is what it is." 'It was what it was,' I told myself. 'Why worry about the past, if even time-traveling won't fix it?'

In a philosophical moment, I reflected on the nature of love. 'If people could see that we all are so similar to one another, they would understand that a relationship with a different partner, who may seem a more perfect match, wouldn't necessarily be better. Why not just love the partner you've got? Isn't he good enough? Wouldn't she just do? If we could believe in lovers' similarity,' I thought, 'so much unnecessary searching, so much heartache would be avoided.'

But at the same time, my romantic self refused to agree with the thesis of similarity. I time-traveled again, this time only in my mind, to a period in my life when I was in the habit of falling in love. Back then, I didn't rely on logic or reason. Like others, I fell in love deep and hard, sometimes too fast. My love was an incurable obsession, pure lunacy. And no matter how much I would call logic or reason into action, there would always remain a part of me which saw my loved one as a singular, unique individual with whom I was destined to live, who I would forever love. In those moments, I was Romeo, in love with my own Juliet, just as Shakespeare had described, and my life couldn't have been saved—not even close.

MY FUNNY BONE

REDHEAD

I fell for a redhead.
She was thin,
and looked the same
from side and front.

She lived in a matchbox,
in the dark, alone.

When I opened the box and entered,
she turned toward me, and said,
'You are so hot!'

I fell for her, did I tell you?
And when I kissed her,
we lit on fire.

She was a perfect match,
the redhead in the box,
and I fell for her.

MY PRIVATE CASE OF MAN FLU

For several weeks, I have been a man wrapped around a painful tooth. My dentist told me that the pain originated in my third, upper molar on the left—my wisdom tooth. "It is technically difficult, perhaps even too late to save the tooth," he said.

Wisdom had to go.

On a Friday afternoon, I lost Wisdom. It took brute force and determination to extract it, for the tooth initially refused to give in. Then, I heard a cracking sound, and *Wisdom* was out.

When my wife, Sharon, returned from work that Friday afternoon, she saw me lying on the sofa under a blanket. On the table beside me were several bottles of medications (antibiotics, pain medicine, and anti-inflammatory drugs) and a glass of water. I was holding a pack of ice over the left side of my face, feeling sorry for myself, moaning and groaning.

"A clear case of the man-flu," she determined without hesitation. "When my wisdom teeth were taken out, all four at once, I took it like a woman!" she added, laughing.

The Oxford dictionary defines "Man flu" as "a cold or similar minor ailment as experienced by a man who is regarded as exaggerating the severity of the symptoms."

The assumption that there is such a thing as "man flu" contributed, in my mind, to the list of other accusations I have heard, on occasion, from the wives of some of my patients. Things like: "men, they never listen," or "men, they never learn," or "men, they don't know what they're talking about."

In an attempt to prove at least one of the accusations wrong (I never learn!), I searched the medical literature. In the light-hearted Christmas issue of the prestigious and very serious *British Medical Journal* (December 2017), I found an article called 'The Science behind "man flu."' It was written by Kyle Sue, an assistant professor in family medicine at the Memorial University of Newfoundland, St John's, Canada.

After he had combed through the medical literature, and methodically reviewed the relevant articles, Kyle Sue reached the following conclusions:

Female mice have stronger immune responses than male mice.

Men (humans this time) with influenza have a higher risk of hospital admission and higher rates of influenza-associated death than women.

These differences extend to respiratory infections other than influenza and to acute diseases affecting the lungs in general; "males are more susceptible to complications and exhibit a higher mortality."

Women are more responsive to the influenza vaccination than men.

As to the behavioral response to the flu, "women were significantly more likely to report cutting down activities in response to only one symptom..."

And, according to an unscientific survey of 2131 readers of a popular magazine, men reported taking an average of three days to recover from viral respiratory illness compared with only 1.5 days for women.

Are the differences between men and women in their response to the common flu real, or does the author's bias play a role? This remains an open question.

If the differences are real, they could be attributed to a deficient immune response in men, differences in the hormonal environment (estrogen in women, testosterone in men), and differences in smoking habits (men smoke more, and smoking is a risk factor for complications from pulmonary diseases).

Perhaps the difference between men and women in their response to the flu is the result of men's "live-hard-die-young" evolutionary strategy. According to this theory, at some point in their evolutionary development, males chose competitiveness and aggressive responses to predators over investing their metabolic resources in a more vigorous immune system (no woman, of course, would fall for such a scheme).

"The concept of man flu, as commonly defined, is potentially unjust," Kyle Sue concludes. Men may not just exaggerate their symptoms, they may experience more severe symptoms. In addition, men's immune systems are weaker and they are prone to greater morbidity and mortality than women.

"Perhaps," Kyle Sue writes, "now is the time for male friendly spaces, equipped with enormous televisions and reclining chairs, to be set up where men can recover from the debilitating effects of man flu in safety and comfort."

Reading all that, I quickly reflected back upon my own condition and the loss of my wisdom tooth. I mumbled a few words of wisdom about evolution and men's vulnerability in the universe (my wife thought I was under the influence of the pain medications). Stretched out on the sofa, I asked my wife to dim the lights and bring me a fresh pack of ice, so that I could recuperate.

And I decided to hold the information I had learned about "man flu" to myself, for I was afraid she would say: "Men! They don't know what they're talking about."

The battle of the sexes, I am telling you, will never end.

WARNING AGAINST JOY

There are warnings everywhere. A label on my toaster announces that I should beware of hot surfaces. My peanut package warns of the possible presence of peanuts inside. And I remember that on a trip to London, at the "Tube" (the underground train), the overhead system constantly reminded me to "mind the gap" (between the platform and the train). Therefore, I was not completely taken by surprise when I read that the universe of warnings has recently expanded to include two human activities that are usually associated with joy.

R. E. Ferner, an honorary professor of clinical pharmacology from the UK, embarked on a mission to explore the benefits and harmful effects of laughter. The results were published in a Christmas edition of the distinguished *British Medical Journal*. Ferner searched the medical literature using the search term 'laugh' and found not less than 4961 scientific articles. Then, articles written by researchers with names such as 'Laughing,' 'Laughter,' and 'Laughton' were removed from the analysis, and so were other articles irrelevant to the subject matter, including research on the Caribbean sponge *Prosuberites laughlini*. After reviewing the remaining articles, Ferner concluded that the potential benefits associated with hearty laughter include decreased anxiety, depression, and anger, as well as a reduced risk of myocardial infarction (heart attack). Examining the potential harms of laughter, the distinguished professor declared that the results were no laughing matter—"Laughter is no joke," he said. The potential complications caused by laughter on the heart, for example, include the development of syncope, cardiac arrhythmias, cardiac rupture, asystolic arrest, and even death. There are also potential negative effects on the respiratory system (triggering an asthma attack, for example), on the central nervous system (leading to cataplexy, the sudden loss of muscle tone, or even a stroke), the gastrointestinal tract, and the urinary tract. It seems that no system in our body is immune to the devastating effects of laughter. The good news, though, is that these severe adverse events have been rare, have usually occurred in patients with medical conditions that made them susceptible to such complications, and have taken place only after an episode of intense and sustained laughter.

Professor Ferner's article itself is entertaining. Reading it, I found myself smiling at first, then giggling, and finally bursting into short episodes of rumbling laughter. In short, I almost fell victim to some of the more serious, harmful effects of laughter, and I feel lucky to be alive!

It seems that laughter is not the only pleasurable human activity that carries rare, yet significant risks, for another article, from the University Department of Emergency Medicine in Bern, Switzerland, suggests that sexual activity may lead to side effects so serious that they require immediate hospitalization. The researchers studied 445 patients that were admitted to the emergency department with medical conditions related to sexual activity. More men than women were injured during sexual activity, and most patients were young. The oldest individuals in the study were a 71-year-old man and a 70-year-old woman. Some patients presented with the usual, expected side effects that are occasionally associated with sexual intercourse—bladder infection, urethritis, and sexually transmitted disease. Others presented with serious complications, such as cardiovascular emergencies or trauma. Head conditions were not uncommon: 27 patients presented with a simple headache, 12 patients had subarachnoid hemorrhage (bleeding into the space surrounding the brain), and 11 suffered from transient global amnesia (perhaps some experiences are better left forgotten). "Sexual activity," the authors claimed, "is mechanically dangerous, potentially infectious, and stressful for the cardiovascular system."

In the sea of warnings around us, one should design a strategy to stay afloat. I ask myself what risks should be ignored, and which risks should be considered an unavoidable cost of participation in the business called life. What actions should we take in order to avoid the risks presented in these articles? Should we wear a frown rather than a smile? Should we suppress even an occasional burst of hearty laughter? Should we be wearing a helmet in the bedroom? To stay afloat in the perpetually expanding sea of warnings, I always mind the gap—the gap between the risks we have come to know and those which are worth avoiding.

DEAR JANE LONEHEART,

You describe yourself as a young woman who is desperately looking for Mr. Right. You have mentioned in your letter that you are looking for a man who is sensitive, spontaneous, and most importantly, someone who possesses "a healthy sense of humor." You also wrote that your mother is encouraging you to marry a doctor, and that you are wondering whether a doctor who is sensitive, spontaneous, and possesses a healthy sense of humor even exists.

Well, Jane, upon reading your letter, I immediately consulted my mental pocketbook of available doctors and found quite a few sensitive and spontaneous doctors who happen to be eligible bachelors. As to whether there is a doctor out there who fulfills the first two requirements and also possesses a healthy sense of humor, I will need to warn you: my answer may be more complex than a simple 'yes' or 'no'!

Perhaps it is best to start discussing humorous doctors by examining the curious case of Dr. Elaine Murphy. One day, back in 1974, she and her husband read a letter, written by Dr. Curtis, to the editor of the prestigious *British Medical Journal*. The letter described three patients—girls learning to play the classical guitar—who developed a condition he called "guitar nipple." According to Dr. Curtis, the inflamed and swollen nipple was the result of the irritation caused by "the edge of the sound box pressed against the nipple." And once the girls stopped playing their beloved instrument, their medical condition, "Guitar Nipple," completely resolved.

The Murphys believed that Dr. Curtis' letter was a prank and decided to retaliate in a humorous way. In a letter to the editor of the same *British Medical Journal*, they described a different condition affecting musicians, and only male musicians: the "cello scrotum." The Murphy letter was not only accepted for publication, it was later cited (together with descriptions of "fiddler's neck" and "flautist's chin") in articles such as "Contact dermatitis and other skin conditions in instrumental musicians."

Please forgive me, Jane, if you found the "cello scrotum" story not especially entertaining, and bear with me, for I have other stories about humorous scientists and physicians. Published bi-monthly, the *Annals of Improbable Research* is a fascinating read for anyone who is interested in scientists and doctors who consider themselves hilarious. The self-described goal of the magazine is to publish research that "makes people laugh and then think." Many of the articles are written in the structured format of a scientific publication, and almost all of them describe an unexpected or absurd experiment, either real or fictional, an experiment that could not be reproduced or should not have been conducted in the first place. The titles of some of the articles are revealing: "Apples and oranges—a comparison," "The effect of television on sexual behavior," and "Does a cat always land on its feet?" In "The sleep-retardant properties of my ex-girlfriend," the author examines the factors influencing his amount of sleep and comes to the conclusion that Hermina, his attractive girlfriend, plays a major role in his sleeplessness. He concludes that he could no longer sleep with Hermina, "an act she termed 'breaking up.'"

The Ig Nobel Prize ceremony at Harvard University is yet another demonstration of awesome scientific humor. At the Ig Nobel Prize ceremony, actual Nobel Prize winners are giving away prizes to other scientists for doing ... strange things. In the Medicine category, for example, the distinguished prize was given for research projects such as: "Acute management of the zipper-entrapped penis," "Injuries due to falling coconuts," and "Termination of intractable hiccups with digital rectal massage." Dan Meyer, the president of the Sword Swallowing Association International, received the 2007 Ig Nobel Prize in Medicine for his investigation of the "Side effects of swallowing swords." He thanked the presenters of the award with a sword still in his throat.

Back to your question, Jane. I do believe there are plenty of sensitive and spontaneous doctors who do possess a healthy sense of humor. But like people in almost any other group of individuals, their sense of humor may be unique and, at times, puzzling to outsiders. Whether you see your potential-husband's medical wit as a good laugh, or see it as a mere "inside joke" depends on your willingness to carefully listen, then understand his frame of mind. Good luck!

SHALL I COMPARE THEE TO A GALAXY?

Scientists warn against comparing apples to oranges. Poets completely ignore their advice.

In a 16-line poem *Introduction to Poetry*, Billy Collins, a former Poet Laureate of the United States, wants you to hold a poem up to the light as if it were a color slide, drop a mouse into a poem as if it were a maze, and waterski across it as if it were a lake. Collins knows that a poem is not a color slide, a mouse maze, nor a lake—he just can't resist the temptation to compare. Poets call these comparisons *similes* and *metaphors*.

In Sonnet 18, William Shakespeare asks: "Shall I compare thee to a summer's day?" He does not wait for permission, for he immediately answers: "Thou art more lovely and more temperate…"

The other day, I felt an intense envy toward poets, and more specifically, for a moment, I just wanted to bathe in their freedom to compare. I decided to take action, and I immediately followed in the footsteps of Shakespeare: "Shall I compare you, My Love, to a galaxy?"

Then, I tried to answer:

The Milky Way, the galaxy that contains our solar system and planet Earth, is of considerable mass. It is about a trillion times bigger than the sun (which itself is two nonillion kilograms). By contrast, at 64 kilograms and 165 cm, you, My Love, are (and I allow myself to be poetic here) not even a speckle of dust. In the *Thee-to-Galaxy Comparison*—and if the bigger the mass, the better—the score is 0:1, with the galaxy winning.

Astronomers use telescopes to observe the galaxy. Lenses, mirrors, and cameras stationed on Earth and in space (the Hubble space telescope, for example) allow scientists to explore the vast universe. On July 4, 2016, after completing a five-year trek, Juno, a spacecraft on a NASA mission, slipped into orbit around Jupiter, the largest planet in our solar system. Juno will allow us to see Jupiter as never before, up close and in spectacular detail. Juno will search for signs of life, as well as rock formations, water, and deep, fast-moving winds. Data and images will be transmitted to Earth.

By comparison, artists, whether they be painters, sculptors, or photographers, would invariably fail to capture your beauty. Doctors might wish to probe deeper in a futile attempt to make sense of your perfect constitution. They might want to use the tools of the astronomers—lenses, mirrors, optic fibers, and digital cameras—to go far and deep in their exploration: ophthalmoscopes to peer into your eyes, otoscopes to closely look at your ear drums, gastroscopes and colonoscopes to survey your intestines, cystoscopes to peer into your bladder, arthroscopes to examine the insides of your knees. I will chase them all away. We will run away to safe harbors.

But how can one compare you to a galaxy without considering the unique building blocks out of which each of you is comprised? The Milky Way contains 100-400 billion stars and 100 billion planets. As to the number of cells in your body, estimates vary, but the most recent estimation puts the number at 37.2 trillion cells. A new analysis published in the journal Cell estimates that an additional 39 trillion bacterial cells live in your intestines. So we have billions of stars and planets measured against trillions of cells and bacteria. The winner is thee, My Love, for you have more components.

You are mortal. The milky way is 13.2 billion years old (I counted). But you, miraculously, can reproduce.

Governed by gravitational forces, stars and planets stay put or move in orbits. The cells in your body, on the other hand, do not just stick to one another to form tissues and organs; they don't just flow in your soupy blood; instead, they function as specialized groups and talk with one another. Hormones that are produced in your pituitary, thyroid, and adrenal glands, for example, command changes in cells throughout your body. Nerve cells in your brain generate tiny electrical circuits and release neurotransmitters that command movements, enable vision, and produce thoughts and feelings, allowing you to become aware of yourself, of me, and of the entire universe. Is a galaxy ever aware of itself? Could a galaxy love me?

"The trouble with poetry," Billy Collins writes, "is that it encourages the writing of more poetry." He adds: "And how will it ever end? Unless the day finally arrives when we have compared everything in the world to everything else in the world."

Shall I compare thee to a galaxy? Perhaps not. But if I had to do it all over again, I would simply conclude: "Thou art more lovely and more temperate . . . "

NEWTON'S APPLE AND MY BIG, RED PLUM

My brother Shlomi was a joker. He was good at telling jokes. I estimate that his inventory included about 50 jokes, short stories with funny punchlines. He would tell, then retell his jokes until I knew them all by heart.

In college, Shlomi took several science classes. This is when he became particularly fond of scientific jokes, short stories with funny punchlines that you could understand only if you had some knowledge of science.

To understand Shlomi's joke about Issac Newton, for example, you needed to know that Sir Issac Newton (1643-1727) was a mathematician and a physicist who laid the foundation for classical mechanics and formulated the laws of motion and the theory of gravitation. To have a good laugh, it wouldn't hurt to know the Apple Incident story, as succinctly told by Voltaire in his *Essay on Epic Poetry*: "Sir Issac Newton walking in his gardens, had the first thought of his system of gravitation, upon seeing an apple falling from a tree." In another version of the story (probably a myth), the apple fell on Newton's head, inspiring him, in a *eureka* moment, to formulate his three Laws of Motion.

To understand Shlomi's joke, you wouldn't need to know the three laws of motion, but, for the sake of completeness, I will briefly remind you of them anyway:

Newton's First Law: Objects in motion tend to stay in motion and objects at rest tend to stay at rest, unless acted upon by an unbalanced force.

Newton's Second Law: Force equals mass times acceleration (F = ma).

Newton's Third Law: For every action there is an equal and opposite reaction.

Now that you know it all, you can easily understand Shlomi's joke. It goes like this:

"Do you know what the three Laws of Newton are?" Shlomi would ask, and just before you would admit that you have no idea, he would jump in and say:

"Here are the three Laws of Newton:

Newton's First Law: The apple doesn't fall far from the tree.

Newton's Second Law: It is good that watermelons don't grow on trees (otherwise the Apple Incident would result in Newton's early demise).

Newton's Third Law: A worm in an apple is better than half-a-worm in half-an-apple (seeing half-a-worm in your apple means that you accidentally ate the other half. Bon Appetit!).

I was reminded of Shlomi's joke late last night. Shai, my son, was back from college for a visit. We were standing in the kitchen. I was eating a big red plum. Before I ate it, I cut the plum into slices. When I was almost done eating, I noticed that the last uneaten slice of the plum had a piece of the price-code sticker still on it.

I showed Shai the slice with the part-sticker and said: "I must have eaten a piece of the bar-code sticker." We laughed for a while, and I said: "It is good that through millions of years of evolution, my body developed the mechanism to overcome such an idiotic mistake."

Shai said, "Yes, perhaps a million years ago, you would have died because of such a mistake. But, it wouldn't have been in vain, for your death would have served the process of natural selection, and future generations would benefit from your misfortune."

"True," I replied, "on the other hand, a million years ago, there wouldn't have been a sticker on my plum."

I found the Plum Incident to be as funny and as revealing as Newton's Apple Incident. It inspired me to think about what makes us laugh. To understand Newton's joke, I would need to know about Newton, the Apple Incident, and the laws of motion. To find the Plum Incident funny, I would have to understand the concept of evolution. In other words, to understand a joke, any joke, one needs to understand the joke-teller's frame of reference.

And in a moment of inspiration, I came upon my own three Laws of Humor (I hope that now that you know my frame of reference, you will find my rules somewhat funny):

Madjar's First Law: Laughter is the best medicine.

Madjar's Second Law: Funny equals sense of humor times shared cultural references (F=SOHxSCR).

Madjar's Third Law: A half-a-price-code-sticker on a half-a-plum is better than a half-a-worm in a half-an-apple.

ACKNOWLEDGEMENTS

I am grateful to my wife, Sharon, who is always a tough critic, but also the most encouraging of readers; to my mother-in-law, Florence, who was instrumental in editing each of the chapters; to my son, Shai, who helped edit the book and added philosophical flavor to some of the stories; and to my sons, Guy and Danny, for giving the book its final illustrative spirit and design.

I am also grateful to Milton Bates, who helped me ease into the world of poetry and gave valuable advice that was tremendously helpful in shaping my poems.

I would like to thank Stacey Willey from Globe Printing, who has helped bring the book to print.

Also, special thanks to the readers of The Mining Journal and The Mining Gazette, whose words of encouragement always motivated me to keep writing.

SHAHAR MADJAR, MD

NOTES ON SOURCES

The Bet
Catron, Mandy L. "To Fall in Love With Anyone, Do This." *The New York Times*, January 9, 2015.

Aron, Arthur, Edward Melinat, Elaine N. Aron, Robert D. Vallone, and Renee J. Bator. "The Experimental Generation of Interpersonal Closeness: A Procedure and Some Preliminary Findings." *Personality and Social Psychology Bulletin 23*, no. 4 (1997), 363-377. doi:10.1177/0146167297234003.

The 25% Desirability Gap
Bruch, Elizabeth E., and M. E. Newman. "Aspirational pursuit of mates in online dating markets." *Science Advances 4*, no. 8 (2018), eaap9815. doi:10.1126/sciadv.aap9815.

A Memorable Read
Wilson, R. S., P. A. Boyle, L. Yu, L. L. Barnes, J. A. Schneider, and D. A. Bennett. "Life-span cognitive activity, neuropathologic burden, and cognitive aging." *Neurology 81*, no. 4 (2013), 314-321. doi:10.1212/wnl.0b013e31829c5e8a.

Eclipse of the Heart
"SIR ARTHUR KEITH (1866-1955) KEITH-FLACK NODE." *JAMA 200*, no. 2 (1967), 164. doi:10.1001/

jama.1967.03120150120031.

Menda, Gil, Paul S. Shamble, Eyal I. Nitzany, James R. Golden, and Ronald R. Hoy. "Visual Perception in the Brain of a Jumping Spider." *Current Biology* 24, no. 21 (2014), 2580-2585. doi:10.1016/j.cub.2014.09.029.

Love by the Numbers

Conley, Terri D., Jes L. Matsick, Amy C. Moors, and Ali Ziegler. "Investigation of Consensually Non-monogamous Relationships." *Perspectives on Psychological Science* 12, no. 2 (2017), 205-232. doi:10.1177/1745691616667925.

Sheff, Elisabeth, and Tikva Wolf. *Stories From the Polycule: Real Life in Polyamorous Families.* Thorntree Press LLC, 2015.

News from Elsewhere... "Japan's 'solo' Weddings." BBC News. Last modified December 22, 2014. https://www.bbc.com/news/blogs-news-from-elsewhere-30574801. Cunard, Nick. "I married myself." *The Guardian,* October 4, 2014

Folie-a-Deux

Nishihara, Ryan, and Craig Nakamura. "A Case Report of Folie'a Deux: Husband-and-Wife." *Jefferson Journal of Psychiatry* 11, no. 1 (1993). doi:10.29046/jjp.011.1.012.

Gorin, Amy A., Erin M. Lenz, Talea Cornelius, Tania Huedo-Medina, Alexis C. Wojtanowski, and Gary D. Foster. "Randomized Controlled Trial Examining the Ripple

Effect of a Nationally Available Weight Management Program on Untreated Spouses." *Obesity* 26, no. 3 (2018), 499-504. doi:10.1002/oby.22098.

La Bella Luna
Redelmeier, Donald A., and Eldar Shafir. "The full moon and motorcycle related mortality: population based double control study." *BMJ,* 2017, j5367. doi:10.1136/bmj.j5367.

The Divorce Party
Staff, AOL. "A Bunch of Celebrities Were Just Spotted Partying at Jeff Bezos' Apartment." AOL.com. Last modified October 31, 2019. https://www.aol.com/article/entertainment/2019/10/31/jeff-bezos-throws-celebrity-packed-party-at-his-nyc-apartment-8-months-after-finalizing-divorce/23850989/.

Dupre, Matthew E., and Alicia Nelson. "Marital history and survival after a heart attack." *Social Science & Medicine* 170 (2016), 114-123. doi:10.1016/j.socscimed.2016.10.013.

Collective Wisdom
Frankovich, Jennifer, Christopher A. Longhurst, and Scott M. Sutherland. "Evidence-Based Medicine in the EMR Era." *New England Journal of Medicine* 365, no. 19 (2011), 1758-1759. doi:10.1056/nejmp1108726.

The Other Girl with the Dragon Tattoo
Coutifaris, Christos, Aoife Kilcoyne, Adam S. Feldman, Mary E. Sabatini, and Esther Oliva. "Case 29-2018: A 31-Year-Old Woman with Infertility." *New England*

Journal of Medicine 379, no. 12 (2018), 1162-1172. doi:10.1056/nejmcpc1807497.

Men are from Earth, Women are from Earth

Gray, John. *Men Are from Mars, Women Are from Venus: Practical Guide for Improving Communication and Getting What You Want in Your Relationships*. New York: HarperCollins, 1993.

Joel, Daphna, Zohar Berman, Ido Tavor, Nadav Wexler, Olga Gaber, Yaniv Stein, Nisan Shefi, et al. "Sex beyond the genitalia: The human brain mosaic." *Proceedings of the National Academy of Sciences* 112, no. 50 (2015), 15468-15473. doi:10.1073/pnas.1509654112.

Of Mice and Men

Stephen M. Walt. "Defending the Indefensible: a How-to Guide." Foreign Policy. Last modified June 2, 2010. https://foreignpolicy.com/2010/06/02/defending-the-indefensible-a-how-to-guide/.

Andres, Young-Mi, Jean-Marc Lassance, Caitlin L. Lewarch, Shenqin Yao, Brant K. Peterson, Meng X. He, Catherine Dulac, and Hopi E. Hoekstra. "The genetic basis of parental care evolution in monogamous mice." *Nature* 544, no. 7651 (2017), 434-439. doi:10.1038/nature22074.

Why is the Y Disappearing?

Meyfour, Anna, Paria Pooyan, Sara Pahlavan, Mostafa Rezaei-Tavirani, Hamid Gourabi, Hossein Baharvand, and Ghasem H. Salekdeh. "Chromosome-Centric Human Proteome Project Allies with Developmental Biology: A Case Study of the Role of Y Chromosome Genes in Organ Development." *Journal of Proteome Research* 16, no. 12 (2017), 4259-4272. doi:10.1021/acs.jproteome.7b00446.

The Rabbit
Blum, Steven M., Morgan L. Prust, Rajesh Patel, Amy L. Miller, and Joseph Loscalzo. "Stream of Consciousness." *New England Journal of Medicine* 378, no. 14 (2018), 1336-1342. doi:10.1056/nejmcps1714950.

Gross, Charles G. "Claude Bernard and the Constancy of the Internal Environment." *The Neuroscientist* 4, no. 5 (1998), 380-385. doi:10.1177/107385849800400520.

My Private Case of Man Flu
Sue, Kyle. "The science behind "man flu"." *BMJ*, 2017, j5560. doi:10.1136/bmj.j5560.

A Warning Against Joy
Ferner, R. E., and J. K. Aronson. "Laughter and MIRTH (Methodical Investigation of Risibility, Therapeutic and Harmful): narrative synthesis." *BMJ* 347, no. dec12 3 (2013), f7274-f7274. doi:10.1136/bmj.f7274.

Pfortmueller, Carmen A., Jana N. Koetter, Heinz Zimmermann, and Aristomenis K. Exadaktylos. "Sexual activity-related emergency department admissions: eleven years of experience at a Swiss university hospital." *Emergency Medicine Journal* 30, no. 10 (2012), 846-850. doi:10.1136/emermed-2012-201845.

Dear Jane Loneheart,

Curtis, P. "Letter: Guitar nipple." *BMJ* 2, no. 5912 (1974), 226-226. doi:10.1136/bmj.2.5912.226-a.

Murphy, J. M. "Letter: Cello scrotum." *BMJ* 2, no. 5914 (1974), 335-335. doi:10.1136/bmj.2.5914.335-a.

www.ingramcontent.com/pod-product-compliance
Lightning Source LLC
Chambersburg PA
CBHW061643040426
42446CB00010B/1559